CONTENTS

Diseases of the vagina

Diseases of the cervix

Diseases of the uterus

Diseases of the fallopian tubes

Diseases of the ovaries

Diseases of the pelvic peritoneum

Diseases of the breasts

PRACTICAL GYNAECOLOGY

With

THERAPEUTIC HINTS

by

Dr. S. P. VERMA
D.H.S. (Hons.)

SECOND REVISED EDITION

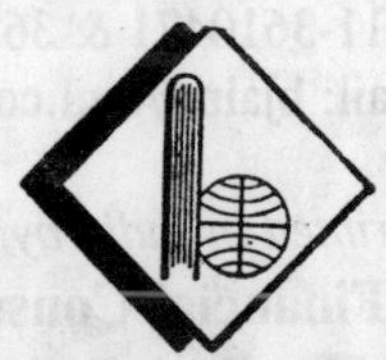

B. Jain Publishers Pvt. Ltd.

NEW DELHI-110055

Price : Rs. 45.00

Reprint Edition: 2001

Published by :
Kuldeep Jain
For
B. Jain Publishers (P.) Ltd.
1921, Street No. 10, Chuna Mandi,
Paharganj, New Delhi 110 055 (INDIA)
Phones: 3670430; 3670572; 3683200; 3683300
FAX 011-3610471 & 3683400
Email: bjain@vsnl.com

Printed in India by:
Unisons Techno Financial Consultants (P) Ltd.
522, FIE, Patpar Ganj, Delhi - 110 092

ISBN 81-7021-197-2
BOOK CODE B-2541

PREFACE

It gives me great pleasure in placing this book before the medical profession.

I noticed the scarcity of the book on this vital subject in the study of medicine for the general practitioners and students, particularly in the field of Homoeopathy. Those, that are available, are meant either for the students or for the practitioners solely, but none that would be beneficial for both. And, in fact, I was inspired by this great need of the medical men. I have collected the best possible available matter on the subject from varied sources for the compilation of this volume. The therapeutic portion has, to a much larger extent, been taken from Drs. Raoue, Guerensey, Wood, Eggert, Dewey, Lilienthal, Boericke and a number of smaller works on the subject; and thus, I have tried to make it useful and worthwhile from every aspect of the study.

To give an account of the superiority of the book would not go to its credit, rather, I feel, it will prove its worth in the mind of the reader when he or she studies it.

In spite of all that, I shall invite and welcome any suggestion from any body for the improvement of the lot in the subsequent editions.

New Delhi. Dr. S. P. VERMA

July 14, 1973.

CHAPTER 1

ANATOMY OF THE FEMALE PELVIS

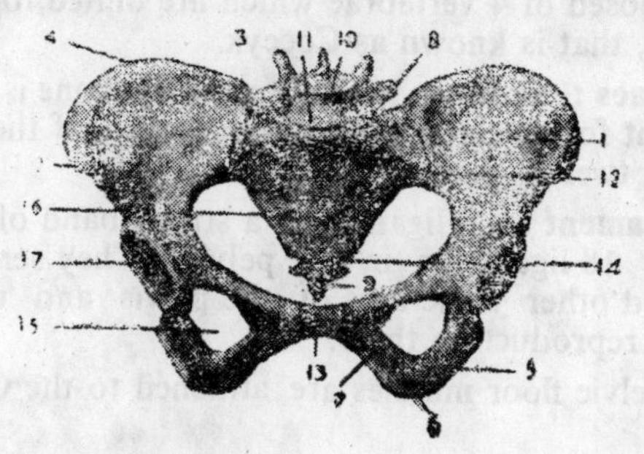

1. Ilium ; 2. Anterior superior spine ; 3. Posterior superior spine ; 4. Crest of the illum ; 5. Ischium ; 6. Tuberosity of the ischium ; 7. Pubes ; 8. Sacrum ; 9. Coccyx ; 10. Fifth lumbar vertebae ; 11. Promontory of the sacrum ; 12. Sacro-iliac joint ; 13. Spmphysis pubis ; 14. Sacro-coccygeal joint ; 15. Obturator foramen ; 16 Foramina for nerves and blood-vessels ; 17. Acetabulum.

PELVIS : is that portion of the body in which the organs of reproduction are contained.

It is composed of the following bones besides other structures :—

1. Innominate bones :—They are two in number situated on either side. Each innominate bone has 3 parts :

(i) Ilium ;

(ii) Ischium ; and

(iii) Pubis.

Ilium is the upper portion. The lower thick portion is called Ischium. And the round shaped portion of it in front has been given the name of Pubis. These are three saparate bones which are fused together in the adult life to make it one bone.

2. Sacrum :—It is, in fact, a part of the vertebral column. Five vertebrae are joined together to form the Sacrum.

3. Coccyx :—It is the last portion of the vertebral column. It is composed of 4 vertebrae which are united together to form one bone, that is known as Coccyx.

4. Spines :—A sharp projection on the bone is called a spine. It is meant for the attachment of ligaments of the pelvis. There are in all, twelve spines, six on either side.

5. Ligament :—A ligament is a strong band of fibrous tissue. There are 18 ligaments in the pelvis. They serve to bind the bones and other structures of the pelvis and to support the organs of reproduction there.

The pelvic floor muscles are attached to the Coccyx behind

— —

CHAPTER II
ORGANS OF REPRODUCTION

For the purpose of description, the female reproductive organs have been divided into external and internal.

EXTERNAL REPRODUCTIVE ORGANS

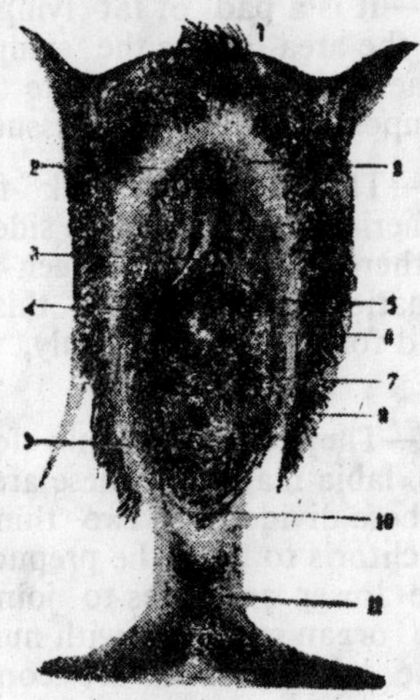

1. Mons veneris : 2. Labia majora ; 3. Clitoris ; 4. Labia minora ; 5. Vestibute ; 6. Urethral orifice ; 7. Orifice of Bartholin's gland ; 8. Vaginal orifice ; 9. Hymen ; 10. Fourchette ; 11. Analorifice.

1. Mons Veneris
2. Labia Majora
3. Labia Minora
4. Clitoris
5. Vestibule

6. Hymen
7. Bartholin's glands
8. Vaginal Orifice
9. Fossa Navicularis
10. Perineum
11. External urethral meatus
12. Mammary glands.

Mons Veneris :—It is a pad of fat lying in front of symphysis pubis. It is the area above the symphysis pubis, i. e., the portion with the hairy growth where pelvic bones join together. It is composed of fibro-fatty tissues.

Labia Majora :—They are two thick folds of the skin inferior to mons veneris, which form the sides of the vulva. It is lobulated, i.e., there is a space between the two. Hernia or Hydrocele formation is possible in this part (but it is a rare possibility, and for this purpose only, its study is important.)

Labia Minora :—They are two thin folds of the skin situated under the labia majora. These are called the inner lips. Anteriorly these divide into two thin folds—the upper one goes over the clitoris to form the prepuce i.e., covering of the clitoris and the lower one goes to join the fraenum. It is a highly sensitive organ supplied with numerous nerves and blood vessels. The labia minora are composed of erectile tissue.

Clitoris :—It is a small body situated at the apex of the labia minora. It is the penis in the female. Like the penis, it has glands, body and crura. Crura joins posteriorly with the pubic bones. It is highly sensitive and consists of erectile tissue.

Vestibule :—It is a triangular shaped space whose apex is formed by Clitoris, base by the anterior margins of the vaginal orifice and the sides are formed by the labia minora.

Hymen :—It is a membrane lying over the vaginal orifice. Previously, its presence was considered to be the sign of virginity ; but, in certain women, hymen is so thin that it is broken with the flow of blood at the time of menstruation ;

while in certain other women, it is so thick hat it is not reptured even at the time of intercourse, it is btroken at the time of child birth only. Therefore, the presence or absence of hymen is not considered to be the sure sign of virginity. But, it is important from the point of view of medical jurisprudence.

Bartholin's Glands :—They are two rounded structures situated on either side of the vaginal orifice in the groove between the hymen and labia minora. They are not palpable until inflamed. Their function is to secrete a sticky secretion under the stimulus of coition for the purpose of lubricating the vagina. They are important because they can be infected and thus get inflamed to which condition we give the name of Bartholinities.

Vaginal Orifice :—It is the opening of the vaginal canal.

Fossa Naicularis :—It means the pit, depression or cavity behind the vaginal orifice.

Perineum :—It is the area between the anus and the vaginal orifice. At the time of delivery, this perineal tear is to be avoided as far as possible.

Urethral Meatus :—It means the external opening of the urethral canal.

Mammary Glands

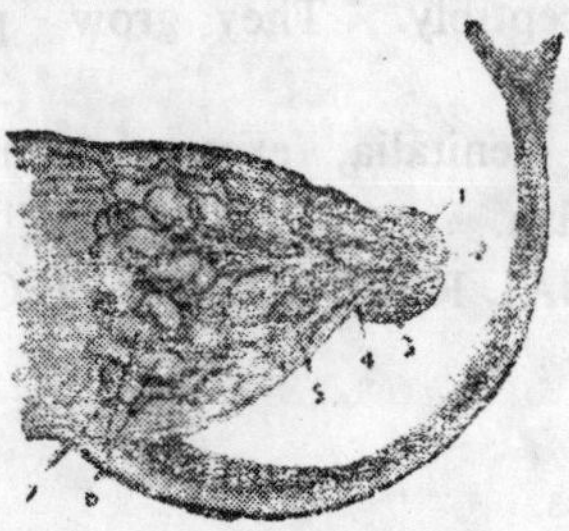

1. Areolā; 2. Nipple; 3, Lactiferous tubule; 4. Ampulla; 5. Lactiferous duct; 6. Lobules; 7. Fat.

They are two in number and are meant to feed the child after birth.

The milk secreting gland or mamma consists of several (15-20) lobules each of which externally resembles a cluster of grapes. The efferent ducts of each lobule open to the exterior in the nipple. When the mamma of a nursing mother is compressed the milk spurts out of the nipple in several thin jets.

In women who have reached sexual maturity the mammae begin to grow perceptibly and the fatty tissue surrounding the individual lobules of the glands develops amply.

The nipple is located in the middle of the breast. Owing to pigmentation the skin of the nipple is of a brownish colour. The nipples differ both in size and shape. A nipple which sufficiently rises above the surface of the breast is considered normal. Flat or retrected nipples are also observed. Subsequently, during pregnancy, it is sometimes possible to eliminate this abnormality by stretching and massage.

The growth of the mammae and the function of the ovaries are very closely interrelated. With the onset of sexual maturity, i.e., when the follicles mature and burst in the ovaries and menstruation appears, the breasts begin to develop quickly and perceptibly. They grow particularly rapidly during pregnancy.

The external genitalia, except mammary glands, as a whole is called Vulva.

INTERNAL REPRODUCTIVE ORGANS

1. Vagina.
2. Uterus.
3. Fallopian tubes.
4. Ovaries.

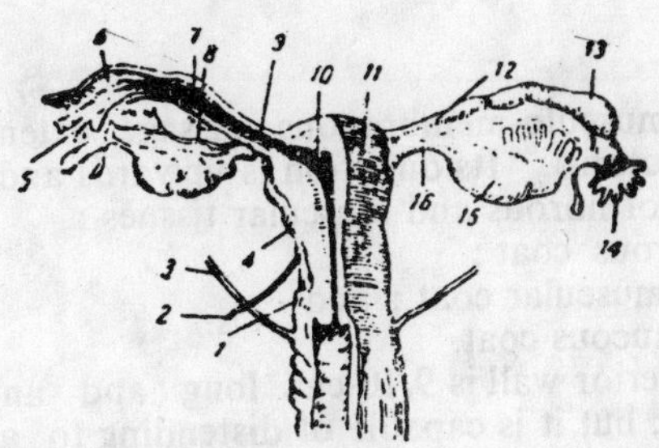

1. Cervical branch of the uterine artery ; 2. Uterine artery ; 3. Ureter ; 4. Ascending branch of the uterine artery ; 5. Fimbriae ; 6. Ampulla of the uterine tube : 7. Isthmus of the uterine tube ; 8. Ovarian vessels ; 9. Interstitial part of the uterine tube ; 10. Uterine cavity ; 11. Peritoneal coat of the uterus ; 12. and 13. Uterine tube ; 14. Ampulla and Fimbriae of the tube ; 15, Ovary : 16. Proper ligament of ovary.

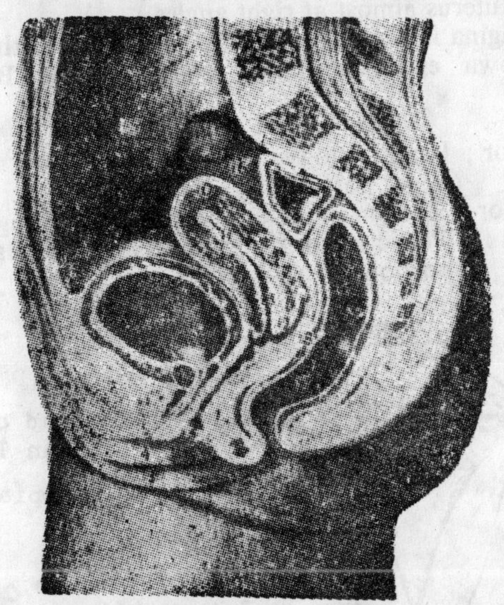

1. Perineal body ; 2. Vagina ; 3. Labia majora ; 4. Labia minora ; 5. Uretha ; 6. Clitoris : 7. Symphysis pubis ; 8. Bladder ; 9. Corpus or body of uterus ; 10. Fundus of uterus ; 11. Cavity of body of uterus ; 12. Cervix or neck of uterus ; 13. Cavity of cervix of uterus ; 14. Abdominal wall ; 15. Abdominal cavity ; 16. Rectum ; 17. Cavity of rectum ; 18. Pouch of Douglas ; 19. Coccyx.

Vagina

It is a musculo-membranous passage extending from the vulva to the uterus. Its direction is upwards and forwards. It is composed of fibrous and muscular tissues :

(i) Outer serous coat ;
(ii) Middle muscular coat ; and
(iii) Inner mucous coat.

Its posterior wall is 9.10 cm. long and anterior wall is 7.8 cm. long ; but it is capable of distending to a considerable extent.

It is located in front of the rectum and at the back of the bladder.

It makes four fornices with the cervix—one anterior, one posterior and two lateral. Porterior fornix is a deeper one on account of the attachment of vagina posteriorly. A fornix is a pocket created by the attachment of vagina with the cervix. It meets the uterus almost at right angles.

The vagina is kept moist by the secretions of the cervical glands, its own epithelial lining and also the Bartholin's glands.

Relations :

Anterior ; Urethra (lower portion) and bladder (upper portion).
Posterior : Rectum, muscles and pouch of Douglas.
Lateral : Pelvic muscles, ligaments and terminal portion of ureters.

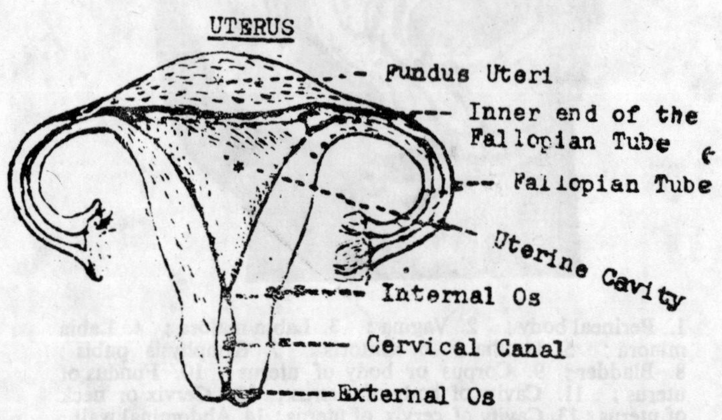

The uterus is placed in the pelvic cavity in the anteverted position between the rectum and the bladder. It consists of :

(i) Outer serous coat ;

(ii) Middle muscular coat ; and

(iii) Inner mucous coat.

It is a hollow organ which is composed of muscles and fibrous tissue—with thick fibro—muscular wall ; inside it are the muscular layer and the endometrium composed of fibrous, muscular and epithelial tissue. Its functions are :

(i) to receive the fertilised ovum ;

(ii) to develop the ovum (baby) and then to expel it at the time of birth ; and

(iii) in its absence, menstruation.

Its shape is like a pear placed in an inverted position.

It is 3″ long (body 2″ and cervix 1″) and has 3l4″ thick wall. (In infants and children, the ratio is body 1″ and cervix 2″).

In an adult woman, weight of the uterus is about 2—1/2 ounces ; but, at the time of full term pregnancy, its weight becomes 2 pounds and after delivery it comes back to almost its normal weight.

Uterus has got 3 parts:—

Body ;

Fundus ; and

Cervix.

Body :—It has a thick fibro-muscular wall and a cavity inside lined by mucous membrane which is known as endomentrium.

Fundus :—It is the upper portion of the body of uterus, i.e. the portion above the entrances of the fallopian tubes. Body and fundus are composed of all the three types of fibrous tissue. It is a highly vasular organ.

Cervix :—It is the lower 1/3 portion of the uterus. It consists of Internal os and External os. It is cylindrical triangular body ; i.e, from the internal os to the external os ; it is cylindrical in shape. The length of the cervical cavity is about 1″.

The direction of the uterus is downwards and backwards. The knowledge of its direction is a great help in locating the different types of displacements of uterus (and also the displacements of the foetus in the uterus).

One layer is around the whole abdominal cavity which is called peritoneum ; and the second layer is around the individual organs of the cbdominal cavity—it is the extension of the peritoneum. In the pelvis, it is called pelvic peritoneum. The uterus forms a pocket like vault in front with the urethra and bladder, which is called Utero-vesical pouch.

Relations :

Anterior : Bladder and utero-vesical pouch.

Posterior : Pouch of Douglas and its contents.

Lateral : Uterine blood vessels, ureters and some ligaments.

Fallopian Tubes :

The are two hollow muscular tubes starting from the upper part of the uterus, called Cornua, and attaching with the ovaries. Each tube is about 4″ in length. They are composed of : (i) Outer serous coat, (ii) Middle muscular layer and (iii) Inner Mucous coat

Function : They carry the ova from the ovaries to the uterus.

Parts :

1. **Interstitial portion**: It is that portion which lies within the uterine wall :
2. **Isthmial portion** : It is the narrow portion lying adjacent interstitial portion :
3. **Ampullary portion** : It is the broad portion of the tube. Conception takes place in this ampullary portion of the tube.
4. **Fimbriaeted portion** : It is the finger like process at the end of the tube. The overlapping fimbriae are called

ovarian-fimbriae they catch hold of the ova from the ovaries when they are released on being matured and thereafter repturing the wall of the ovary.

Ovaries :

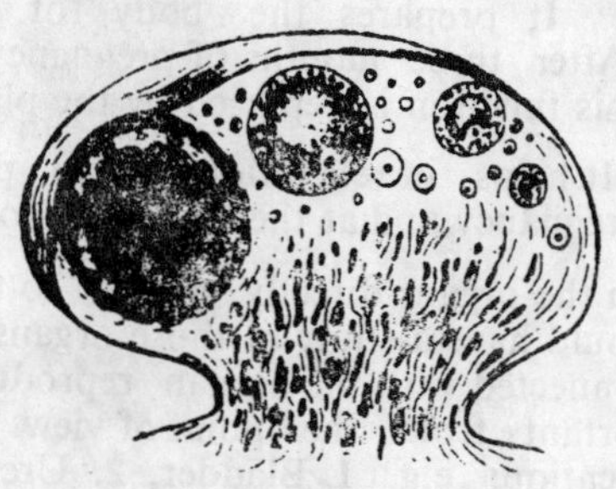

They are two in number placed in the lateral walls of the pelvis on either side of the uterus.

Size : The ovary is an almond shaped organ. In an adult female, it is about 1½″ long, ½″ thick and 3/4″ in depth.

In the ovaries, there are numerous small cystic spaces, known as Graffian follicles, containing ova in them; some of them are ripe or mature, while others are immature. There are about 70,000 Graffian' follicles ; but only one of them matures every month (12 in a year and about 360 in whole of the menstrual life of a woman if she does not get fertilised or impregnated at all). When the ovum becomes mature, it ruptures the wall of the ovary and escapes out of the peritoneal cavity. Then the fallopian tube catches hold of the ovum and conveys it to the uterus.

Functions : (1) To produce the ovum, and (2) To secrete hormones—(i) Oestrin, (ii) Progesterone, and (iii) Relaxin.

Oestrin :—It is secreted by the Graffian follicle. It controls the activities of the uterus and the breasts throughout the menstrual cycle and pregnancy.

Progesterone :—When the Graffian follicle ripens, it ruptures its wall and throws out the ovum. At the site of the ruptured place a new substance is formed; this new substance is called Corpus Luteum and is yellow in colour. Progesterone is the hormone secreted by the Corpus Luteum (Corpus Luteum is a latin word : Corpus means body and Luteum means yellow). It prepares the body for pregnancy after conception. After three months of pregnancy, its secretion is stopped and this function is replaced by the placenta.

Relaxin:—It helps in relaxation of the pelvic organs and ligaments in pregnancy and at the time of labour.

Apart from the organs directly related to the reprodructive system, we should have a study of those organs also which are not directly connected with the human reproduction, but their study is important from the point of view of avoiding any serious complication; e.g. 1. Bladder, 2. Urethra, 3. Ureters, and 4. Rectum.

Urinary Bladder :—It is placed in front of the uterus.

Relations : 1. Anterior—Pubic bone.
2. Posterior—Uterus and utero-vesical pouch; base of the bladder is related to cervix.

Urethra :—It is a passage of urine from the bladder to the exterior. Its length is about 1½″.

Relations : It is in close contact with the anterior vaginal wall. At the time of delivery, there may be perforation of the vaginal wall injuring the urethra also. It can be dilated with ease upto 1″, because the foreign body of that length has been found passing through it.

Ureters :—They are two tubes running on either side from the kidneys to the bladder. Each measures about 12″ in length. Their lower portion is lying closely with the cervix. Their situation is very important from the surgical point of view, because at the time of operation, they may get ruptured. It is important from the medical point of view as well, because certain disease or any inflammation may compress them causing uraemia.

Rectum :—It is the end portion of large intestine which has three portions—aecum, Colon and Rectum. It starts from 1″

away from the tip of the Coccyx. In the middle of the rectum, it takes the curve laterally towards the left. It is important for the purpose of enema and introduction of any instrument.

R*elations* :

Anterior : Pounch of Douglas, lower portion of it is in relation with the posterior wall of vagina and cervix.

Posterior : Sacral vertebrae.

Lateral : Ligaments.

CHAPTER III

LIGAMENTAL ATTACHMENT

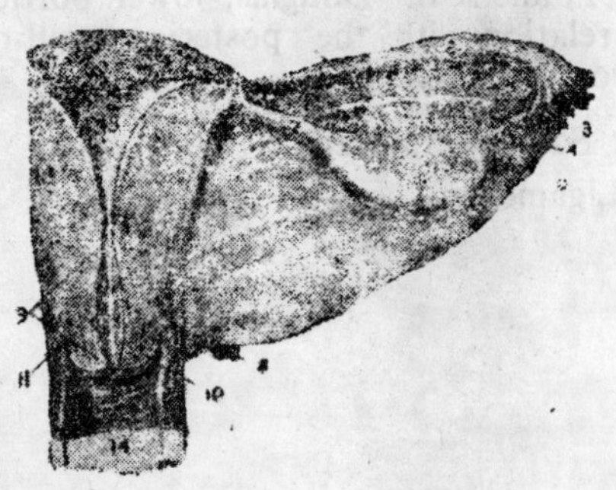

1. Duct of Gartner; 2. Fallopian tube; 3. Ampullary opening; 4. Hydatid of Margagni; 5. Round ligament, Ovarian vassels; 6. Ovary; 7. Ligament of ovary; 8. Ureter; 9. Neck of uterus ; 10. Vaginal portion of neck of uterus ; 11. Laterāl fornices of vagina; 12. body of uterus; 13. Cavity of uterus ; 14. Vagina.

Ligaments are of two varieties :—

A. Accessory ligaments, and

B. Real or true ligaments.

A. ACCESSORY LIGAMENTS

They do not keep the healthy uterus in position, but, they do form the pelvic floor binding other structures of the pelvis, e.g. bones, etc. They are as follows :—

1. Broad ligament. It is a double fold of the peritoneum running laterally and slightly backward from the uterus. From above and front, it is continuous with the side walls of the pelvis and here, it is known as **Infundibulo—pelvic ligament.** Ovary divides this ligament into two parts :—

(i) Upper part, called Meso-salpinx, and
(ii) Lower part, named Parametrium which contains some important structures, like blood vessels, neves, lymphatics, etc., in between the two layers.

Meso-salpinx contains :

(a) Fallopian tubes (b) Broad ligament
(c) Ovarian ligament (d) Par-ovarian
(e) Branches of ovarian and uterine arteries anastomosing there.

Parametrium contains :

(a) Ureters
(b) Uterine vessels
(c) Lymphatic glands
(d) Lymphatic duct (Gartner's duct)
(e) Cellular tissue.

2. **Round ligament :**—It is a slender cord like structure which comes from each cornua long the anterior layer of broad ligament through internal abdominal ring (where hernia takes place), inguinal canal and external abdominal ring to the labium major on each side.

3. **Utero-sacral ligament :**—It is on the posterior surface of the uterus and forms the pouch of Douglas in between the uterus and secrum.

4. **Overian liagment :**—It also comes from the cornua and is attached to the ovaries.

B. **True Ligaments.**

The uterus and bladder are kept in position chiefly by three fascial layers—two are horizontal and one is vertical. These layers contain unstriate muscles as well as fascia, known as :

1. **Orchus tendnusfaci pelvic.** It passes from symphysis pubic to ischial spines with extension to sacrum.

2. **Lateral pelvo-vesicular ligament :**—It arises from the pelvis on each side and embraces the neck of the bladder, upper part of the vagina and isthmus of the uterus.

3. **Cardinal ligament of the Cervix.** It passes from one ischial spine to another and sets about vertically in the erect posture.

Blood and Nerves :

Branches from the Internal iliac artery supply the blood to the uterus and anastomose there on each side.

Nerve supply to the uterus is from the sacral and lumbar plexus.

CHAPTER VI
BLOOD SUPPLY TO PELVIC ORGANS

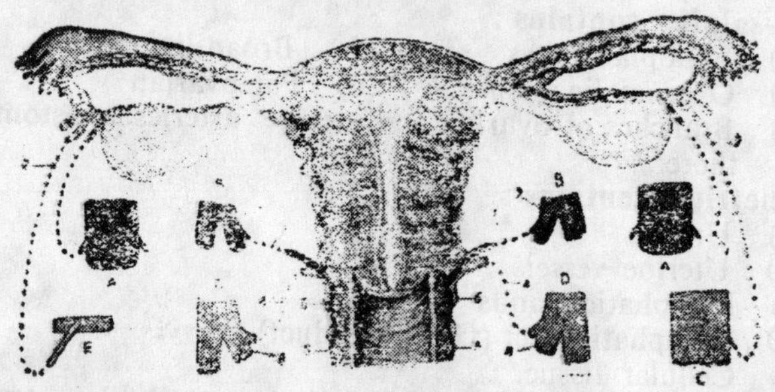

1. Ovarian artery. 2. Ovarian vein. 3. Uterine artery. 4. Uterine vein. 5. Vaginal artery. 6. Veginal vein. 7. Internal iliac artery. 8. Internal iliac vein.

A. Aorta. B. Common iliac artery. Inferior vena cava. D. Common iliac vein. E. Left renal vein.

The blood which is coming from the heart to different parts of the body is fresh blood and is called the arterial blood supply.

And the blood coming from different parts of the body to the heart is deoxygenated and is known as the venous blood supply.

Biggest blood vessel in the body is Aorta ; it is further divided and subdivided into arteries, arterioles and finally capillaries.

Aorta :

(i) Ascending aorta.
(ii) Arch of aorta.
(iii) Decending or thoracic aorta.
(iv) It goes further and enters the abdominal cavity where it is called the abdominal aorta.
(v) Right and left coronary arteries supply the blood to the heart muscles.
(vi) Innominate artery.

(vii) Left and right common carotid arteries.
(viii) Left and right subclavian arteries.

Abdominal aorta is further divided into eight parts. One of these arteries further divides into two common—iliac arteries ; each again is divided into two which supply blood to the legs :

(a) Right external common iliac artery,
(b) Right internal common iliac artery, and
(a) Left external common iliac artery.
(b) Left internal common iliac artery.

PELVIC ORGANS :

1. Ovarian artery :—Its source is abdominal aorta. It bifurcates into two, each one going to the ovaries and fallopian tubes

2. Internal iliac artery :—It starts from the bifurcation of abdominal aorta and divides into Anterior and Posterior trunks and further divides into eight branches, four of which are supplying blood to the pelvic organs.

(i) Uterine artery : supplying blood to the uterus
(ii) Vaginal artery : supplying blood to the vagina.
(iii) Middle vesical artery : supplying blood to the lower and lateral portions of bladder.
(iv) Superior vasical artery : supplying blood to the upper portion of bladder.

3. Superior haemorrhoidal artery:—It supplies blood to the rectum.

System of arteries :—Aorta, arteries, arterioles and finally a net-work of capillaries.

System of veins :—Out of the net-work of capillaries, smaller veins originate ; they meet into bigger veins, then still bigger veins and finally the biggest veins, Inferior-venacava bringing blood from lower portion of the body and Superior-venacava bringing blood from upper portion of the body. All the deoxygenated blood will go to inferior and superior venacavae.

System of venous blood from pelvic organs to inferior venacava

1. Vesical plexus	from	bladder
2. Rectal plexus	from	rectum
3. Uterine plexus	from	uterus
4. Vaginal plexus	from	vagina
5. Ovarian veins	from	ovaries.

CHAPTER V
ENDOCRINAL PHYSIOLOGY

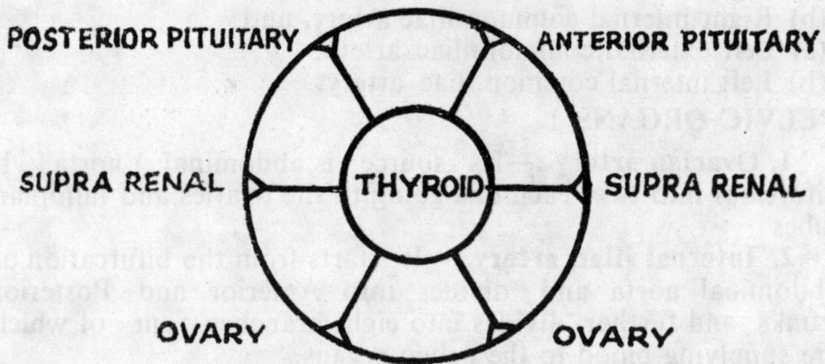

A. Thyroid Gland

It is intimately related to genital organs and functions in the following ways :—

(i) It enlarges at puberty, before menses and during pregnancy.

(ii) It is more liable to disease in women. Exophthalmic goitre is often associated with menorrhagia in early states and myxoedema with amenorrhoea.

(iii) It apparently aids nidus of ovum ; hence its use inhabitual abortionsis recommended.

(iv) Thyroid secretion accelerates involution and aids lactation.

(v) Hyposecretions may cause under development of uterus, especially, in regard to musculature, causing severe dysmenorrhoea. (If such cases are treated with thyroid and ovarian extracts before they reach 20 years, the result is usually satisfactory).

(vi) Hyperthyroidism between 18 and 24 years of age often causes menorrhagia.

B. Posterior Pituitary Gland.

(i) It increases in size during pregnancy and after Cophorectomy.

(ii) It produces oxytocin and vaso-pressin-(hormones that press the blood vessels).

(iii) The oxytocic hormone causes contraction of the uterus after 6th month of pregnancy and in early puerperium (lying period after delivery) ; but, its action is very slight before that time. In fact, in the very early months, it may cause relaxation rather than contraction.

C. Anterior Pituitary Gland

(i) It governs menstrual cycle through ovaries.

(ii) When it is removed, the ovaries get atrophied and oestrin is completely suppressed, whereas the grafting of anterior pituitary gland re-establishes these functions.

(iii) Castraction of anterior pituitary causes increase in size and function of the overies. Subsequently, that one of the ovarian hormones has inhibiting effect, probably that is oestrin.

(iv) Hyposecretion causes dwarfism (short stature), hypophyscal cachexia (this is knows as Simmond's disease).

(v) Hypersecretion causes giantism (huge size) and acromegaly (having a large face),

(vi) Probably, it produces hormones causing milk-secretion.

D. Supra Renal Glands

(i) They enlarge during pregnancy.

(ii) Removal of one causes some atrophy of the uterus, but the pregnancy is not interfered with.

(iii) Excessive secretion causes sterility and amenorrhoea with loss of feminine characteristics.

(iv) They cause retention of calcium salts acting contrary to thyroid activity.

E. Thymus

(i) It atrophies at puberty owing to the function being taking over by the ovaries.

(ii) A persistent thymus is often accompanied by amenorrhoea and defective genital organs.

F. Ovaries

Two distinct hormones are secreted by the ovaries : One is derived from the Graffian follicle, that is Oestrin and the other from the Aorpus Luteum, that is Progesterone. Oestrin causes enlargement and increased vacularity of the uterus : whereas progesterone inhibits ovulation and sensitises the endometrium to receive the fertilized ovum. It also causes the premenstrual changes in the uterus. During pregnancy, progesterone aids the nourishment of the ovum until the placenta is formed and inhibits the uterine contractions. Oestrin, on the other hand, promotes the uterine contractions and inhibits the conception. Anterior lobe of the pituitary gland produces probably two hormones which act on the ovaries ; Prolan--A evokes oestrin and Prolan--B which causes luteinization with the formation of progesterone. Prolan--A is found in large quantity in the urine of pregnant women, greatest amount being present at the 5th month of pregnancy after which the quantity gradually diminishes ; whereas the quantity of oestrin excreted in the urine is greatest at the end of pregnancy. Thus, injection of urine from pregnant women which contains a large quantity of Prolan--B causes luteinization of the follicles if injected into the immature female mice causing a blood-spot to appear and this fact has been proved by Aschheim and Zondek in their tests for the confirmation of pregnancies. A correct result has been obtained in over 98% of cases after one period is missed.

CHAPTER VI

MENSTRUATION

Menstruation is also called menses or monthly period in the common layman language.

It means the periodic flow of blood from the uterus after 28 days on an average, the range being 24 to 32 days, as a result of haemorrhagic destruction of the endometrium due to non-fertilization of the ovum. The flow usually persists for 3-5 days and the amount of blood lost during the period is about 2-8 ounces.

The usual age of occurance is between 12—14 years ; it is slightly earlier in hot countries or short statured girls.

Alongwith the menses, there are certain other changes also ; e.g , enlargement of breasts, thyroid and parotid glands ; in fact, these glands get enlarged at puberty. At that time, the woman usually gets acnes, and some laziness also. Lassitude and headache are common features. As regards pulse. it is diminished in rate. Blood pressure is raised in premenstrual stage and is lowered after the flow starts. R.B.Cs are increased in premenstrual stage and decreased after the flow. Coagulation of blood is diminished during the period ; so, care, should be taken to avoid injury. There is a rise in the calcium index in the blood and more calcium is passing in the blood flow. The contents which are passed with the blood are:—

(i) Mucin =33%

(ii) Lactic acid

Epithelial cells are destroyed. As nofibrin is present, so, the blood does not clot. Clot is an abnormality.

Theories about Menstuation

There are different theories which have been put forward for the occurance of menstruation.

1. It is the preparation for the fertilized ovum during the menstrual period. When fertilization does not take place the ovum comes out of the uterus.

2. It is due to blood borne secretions from the ovaries. If the ovaries are removed and transplanted; menstruation goes on and it consists of shedding from the uterus of tissues prepared for the fertilized ovum.

3. It is due to internal secretions of the ovary and not on account of ovulation. (Pregnancy may take place before menses occur during lactation and also at times after menopause). Ovulation may also occur during periods of secondary amenorrhoea.

4. Calcium content of the blood is very high before the menses ; that menstrual blood has a high calcium content and the calcium content in general circulation falls rapidly during menses.

5. Anterior pituitary hormone evokes oestrin from Graffian follicle which ruptures and luteinization occurs. The corpus luteum produce an excess of oestrin besides progesterone ; and this excess of oestrin inhibits the anterior pituitary causing regression of corpus luteum with sudden cessation of oestrin which produces menses. Removal of corpus luteum at operation is followed by meness in 2 days.

Physiology of Menstruation

The changes occuring in the uterus are called the endometrial cycle ; and the changes occuring side by side in the ovaries are called the ovarian cycle.

This all is under the control of anterior pituitary gland. Menstruation is divided into 4 phases (starting from the first day) :—

1. Bleeding and rapair of the uterine lining : Ist to 7th day.
2. Growth of the uterine lining ; 7th to 12/13th day.
3. Ovulation : around 14th day.
4. Congestion of the uterine lining and other preparations 14th-28th day.

During the first 7 days, i. e., first phase, the anterior pituitary gland secretes a hormone, known as follicle stimulating hormone -- (F.S.H.) which acts upon the ovaries and make them secrete another hormone—oestrin. Oestrin circulates in the blood and acts upon the uterus ; and under the action of oestrin, old uterine lining is stripped off and a new lining is formed.

In the second phase, the new lining grows and shows regeneration side by side, in the ovaries one ovum ripens in the graffian-follicle, and it comes nearer the surface of the ovary. The folliele is filled with the fluid also.

In the third phase, on or about the 14th day, the graffian follicle ruptures and the ovum is freed from the ovary ; it is known as ovulation. The action of F.S.H. is upto 14th day.

In the last phase, i. e. from 14th to 28th day, another hormone, luteinizing hormone (L.H.), is secreted by anterior pituitary gland. It acts upon the ovaries causing a membrane to form on the ruptured surface of the graffian—follicle which is yellow in colour and known as Corpus Luteum. This new structure secretes another hormone known as progesterone. It circulates in the blood and acts upon the uterus making it spongy, soft, thick and calm At this stage, the uterus is fully prepared to receive the fertilized ovum.

If pregnancy does not take place, the same cycle is repeated.

In this way, menstruation has also been defined as "weeping of the uterus for the destruction of unfertilized ovum."

If pregnancy takes place, corpus luteum persists which keeps the uterus calm and quite ; after that, this function is taken over by the placenta.

Ovular Menstruation

It is the one which contains the ovum in it and is associated with all the changes that take place in the endometrium under the influence of the ovarian hormones—oestrin and more particularly progesterone. It is present during whole of the child bearing age, i.e., from puberty to menopause.

Anovular Menstruation

It is the menstruartion which does not contain the ovum in and it is not associated with the progestational changes in the endometrium. The menstruation is there alright ; but, the progestational changes would not be present in the en·dometrial lining of the uterus. So, it is very difficult to make a clinical differentiation between an ovular menstruation and an anovular menstruation.

The D & C (dilatation and curettage) operation is performed and the uterine lining is scraped and these scrapings are sent to the laboratory for microscopic examination for the presence of progestational changes. This type of menstruation is met within sterile women or in women near the climacteric. It may be due to some defect of the ovaries or the pituitary gland itself.

And their significance in the treatment

The right knowledge of the disease leads us to adopt the correct line of treatment, otherwise, we shall meet failure. If the underlying disease or condition is such without the removal of which the patient's sufferings cannot be eliminated and the treatment is continued on wrong lines, the result will be utter disappointment on the part of the patient and the physician also. Say, for example, if the ovaries are diseased, such as cystic changes, unless the underlying defect is treated and corrceted, brilliant results cannot be expected.

——

CHAPTER VII

SOME COMMON REMEDIES

In this chapter, some of the common remedies, which generally come to our mind, for the different affections of the women, have been given. These are not the only remedies to be thought of; there are a number of other remedies as well, depending upon the symptoms. The symptoms from the basis of our prescription, whatever the disease may be.

Aletris farinosa :—The key note symptom here is "tired all the time." The menses are early and profuse with labour like pains. Useful in uterine displacements and leucorrhoea, when attended by extreme constipation and weak digestion. Suppressed menses, when the patient is nervous, hysterical and sleepless. She is tired, dull, heavy, unable to concentrate the mind on anything. Tired feeling, extreme constipation and weakness of digestion; it is the trinity of this remedy.

Belladonna :– Bearing down, worse lying down and better by standing. Menses are profuse and early, of bright red blood. with cramps in back and arms. Dysmenorrhoea with cutting pains through the pelvis in a horizontal direction ; the pains are paroxysmal and the discharge is often offensive. Metritis, with sensation of heat and great sensitiveness, and bearing down. In all the acute inflammations of the pelvic organs, where the pains are severe, clutching and throbbing, more on right side, worse by the slightest jar.

Calcarea Carb :—The menses are abnormal, being early and profuse and lasting too long, with cold and damp feet. Amenorrhoea, especially the first menses are delayed, and these are apt to be, as a result, congestion to the head or chest, haemorrhage, night cough, general anaemia and unnatural appetite. Leucorrhoea is milky, at times profuse, with itching and burning. The peculiar constitution is, of course, not to be ignored ; that is, fat, fair and flabby ; the craving for chalk, mud and other indigestible things, etc.

Cimicifuga :—The patient is gloomy and full of dejection ; has a sensation as if she would go crazy. Early and profuse menses, attended with wandering pains in the back. Dysmenorrhoea with an irritable, sensitive bruised uterus and pains flying across the hypogastrium from side to side. Leucorrhoea, when present with nervousness, neuralgic pains and hyperaesthesia. Sensation of weight in the uterus. Sharp shooting pains in the ovaries with a bearing down sensation. Facial blemishes, acne, rough skin in young girls at menstrual periods. Apart from these symptoms, there are headache and rheumatism affecting the muscles.

Ferrum Iod :—Pale, anaemic, scrofulous patients Prolapsus uteri with bearing down pains in the pelvis, and a feeling as if the uterus descended so as to be pushed up when sitting. Starchy leucorrhoea. Pressure on the rectum. Menses are more painful than usual.

Helonias :—Atony of the genital organs and pain from the back to the uterus. "Consciousness of the womb" is a keynote symptom ; with constant soreness and weight in the womb accompanied by a tired, aching felling in the back and limbs. Leucorrhoea dark, offensive, and constant ; it flows on every exertion. General debility and pruritus may be present. Often indicated in vaginitis and vulvitis ; the mucous membrane is red, inflamed and itching is intense. Too frequent and profuse menses and the flow is dark, coagulated and offensive. Abortion from the slightest over-exertion and sterility due to great debility Displacements of the uterus with heaviness in hypogastirum, a tired, dragging feeling in the back, extending all over the body upon slight exertion.

Kreosote :—The menses are profuse, with humming and roaring in the head and preceded by abdominal bloating ; the flow may be intermittent and accompanied with drag ing downwards in the back. Dark brown and offensive leucorrhoea often following the periods ; it is very acrid, very offensive and excoriating ; it is yellow, the patient is weak, there is violent itching of the vagina and smarting and burning between the thighs. The parts become swollen, hot, hard and sore. Prolapsus uteri with dragging in the back, and a dragging downward which are relieved by motion. Ulcerations about the genital organs, with offensive excoriating discharge, burning pain, heat and soreness.

Lilium Tig :—Leucorrhoea is watery, yellow or yellowish-brown and excoriating. There is much nervousness and aimless burning ; the mind and body are weak and the patient lacks confidence. Useful in uterine symptoms following pregnancy and labour. when the uterus is heavy has not regained its normal size, nor returned to its normal position; so there is heavy dragging in the hypogastrium, which is relieved by moving about. There is urging for urination and stool with sexual excitement. It has violent ovarian pains especially of the left side, shooting down anterior and inner side of the thigh.

Platina :—Here, the mental symptoms decide the choice ; the pride, the haughtiness, the self-esteem and the belitting of everyone ; then also, the strange feelings in which the home objects seem un-familiar · also, the melancholy. Menses are profuse and clotted and occur early, with nymphomania. Induration and prolapse of the uterus, with continual pressure in the groins and back. Also for painful intercourse. Chronic induration of the ovaries. Oophoritis with burning pains and numbness of the limbs.

Pulsatilla :—This is the first remedy coming in our mind for the treatment of diseases of the women. Dysmenorrhoea : scanty, and delayed menses with severe griping pains, sometimes compelling her to double up. Amenorrhoea ; the menses flow by fits and starts, due to wetting of the feet, and also delayed menses in chlorotic girls. Leucorrhoea is usually thick, creamy or milky, but it may be thin acrid and associated with swelling of the vulva, worse before menses, and accompanied by delayed and scanty menses. With all these symptoms, the Pulsatilla temperament is always present ; i.e., gentleness, timidity, mildness, even tearfulness, also fickleness, indecision and changeableness.

Secale Cor :—Uterine haemorrhage; with a passive, painless flow of dark fluid blood, worse by motion. Wrinkled, scrawny women, who become cold and formication is present.

Sepia :—Menses usually late and scanty and dark, but may be early and scanty or early and profuse, accompanied by discolouration of the skin, preceded by aching in abdomen and colicky pains. Amenorrhoea, with the Sepia temperament where there is extreme sensitiveness to all impressions.

Leucorrhoea yellow-green in colour and somewhat offensive ; but may be milky also ; worse before menses and accompanied by bearing down. Uterus is found to be enlarged and cervix indurated ; a useful remedy in displacements, especially prolapse and retroversion, with irritability of bladder and lecorrh ea. Bearing down pains with a feeling as if everything would protrude from the vulva, relieved by sitting with the legs crossed ; with lumbo-sacral backache. Great dryness of the vulva and vagina ; painful to touch- hence its usefulness in dyspareunia Chronic Oophoritis, with dull, heavy pains and other Sepia symptoms. Weakness, sallowness, epigastric goneness and heaviness are great characteristics. Yellow complexion, the yellow saddle over the nose, the sunken dark-ringed eyes, the relief from violent motion and in the middle of the day ; and general want of tone in the whole body are great indications. Lack of affection which develops in the mind is most importent mental symptom.

Zincum Valeriana :—It has restlessness, with nerve fag from ovarian and uterine irritation, long continued anxiety, and loss of rest from care of the children. The uterus is heavy, but the ovaries are highly tender. It suits quick fidgety nervous women easily fagged out with aching, sensitive ovaries.

There are some other remedies which require consideration : Aconite, Ammon. Carb., Apis Mel., Bellis Per., Bovista, Carbo Veg , Caulophyllum, Causticum, Chaomilla, China, Coccus Cacti, Conium. Dulcamara, Erigeron, Ferum Fraxinus Americana, Hamamelis, Iodine, Ipecac, Magnesia Phos., Millefolium, Murex, Natrum Mur., Palladium, Phosphorus, Sabina. Senecio Aureus, Silicea, Sulphur, Trillium, Ustilago, etc., etc.

—.—

CHAPTER VIII

STERILITY AND DYSPAREUNIA

STERILITY

Definition :—Sterility means difficult or no conception; to be more clear, it is the inability on the part of the male or the female partner to produce any offspring.

Conception depends upon the normal development and functions of the genitalia and sexual organs of both the female and the male, in addition to proper mating. Any defect, temporary or permanent, in either male or female partner leads to sterility. The examination should be conducted to find out the cause. The woman is, however, more often found unproductive; but, in certain cases (about 25% of sterile cases), the male is also defective; so the husband must not be forgotten. The poor women, and innocent girls, sometimes. have to undergo operations unnecessarily, while the fault lies with the husband.

Causes in Females

In females, the causes of sterility may be divided into two groups — :

A. Ceneral, and

B. Local.

A. General Causes

1. Nerotic : hystenia, indifferences and other mentel conditions.
2. Debilitating diseases like anaemia, tuberculosis, causing amenorrhoea and scanty menstruation.
3. Endocrinal deficiencies : obesity due to defective thyroid secretion.
4. Incompitibility between husband and wife.

B. Local Causes

1. Absence of any essential part of the genitalia; e.g., removal of uterus, tubes or ovaries.
2. Atresia of cervix and rudimentary uterus.
3. Imperforate hymen : (can be cured by minor operation).
4. Pinhole os causing mechanical obstruction to spermatozoa. (It can be cured by simple dilatation which may not be lasting).
5. Hypertrophy of the cervix : Operative treatment is essential here, and that is amputation of the vaginal portion of the cervix.
6. Malformation or destruction of tubes—due to inflammatory conditions like gonorrhoeal salpingits, appendicitis, etc. (If the lining membrane of the tube is affected, the sterility would be absolute).
7. Partial stenosis of the tubes: it is associated with imperfectly developed uterus (almost an incurable condition).

Rubin's Test

It is performed to see whether the tube is potent or not, blocked or permeable. In this test, air or carbon dioxide is passed into the uterus by Rubin's apparatus through the cervix under slight pressure (Cervix is dilated first under anaesthesia). The air or gas should pass easily through the tube into the abdomen in a normal and potent tube. We can hear the air entry by stethescope. But, if a pressure greater than 200 mm is required, some tubal obstruction is diagnosed. Greater pressure than 200mm should not be used for the danger of bursting of the tube.

Another way of test of the potency and permeability of the tubes is by the introduction of a dye (lipoidol), injected into the uterus ; a subsequent X—ray will show not only that the tubes are blocked or n t, but also the sites where they are blocked.

This test is for diagnostic as well as curative purposes ; because, in some cases, lipoidol clears the obstruction.

8. Inflammatory conditions : such as endometritis, endocrevicitis.
9. Cystic ovaries or destroyed as well, due to tumours etc.
10. Vaginismus : It means the painful and spasmodic reflex contraction of the muscles surrounding the vaginal orifice during coitus, and during digital examination. So, intercourse is not possible. It may be due to the following reasons :—

    (i) Nervousness and hysteria;

    (ii) Smallness of vulva and vagina-congenital or acquired; and

    (iii) Inflammatory conditions.

    Ars., *Bell.*, *Cup.*, and *Mag.*, *Phos.* often prove beneficial in this condition if the symptomatology corresponds.
11. Displacement of uterus :

    (i) Retroversion may cause sterility by tilting the cervix so far forwards that spermatozoa find it difficult to enter the uterus.

    (ii) Prolapse of the uterus may prevent coitus.

    (iii) Chronic inversion : the uterus is inverted from within outwards.
12. Trauma to the parts : laceration of cervix with evertion causing a discharge which may prevent ingress of spermatozoa.
13. New growths—fibroids and cancer, etc.

In Males :

1. Impotency.
2. Some developmental defect : e.g., short and curved penis, hypospadias, undescended or strophied testes, etc.
3. Defective seminal disharges : no sperms or undeveloped sperms or a few sperm non-motile sperms; this may be due to some previous or present disease of the testes, like mumps, tuberculosis, gonorrhoea, syphilis, etc.

Investigations in Male :

1. Compatibility of husband and wife.
2. General condition and development of genital organs.

3. Examination of semen for the presence and motility of the spermatozoa.

In Female

A. General physical examination, and

B. Local examination.

A. General Physical Examination

1. State of menses; menorrhagia, metrorrhagia, dysmenorrhoea or scanty menstruation.
2. General state of health; good or poor, anaemia etc.
3. Debilitating diseases; like tuberculosis.
4. Venereal diseases; e.g. syphilis and gonorrhoea.
5. Urine for albumin and sugar.

B. Local Examination

1. Congenital defects of the genitalia; like;

Vagina :—Imperforate hymen, tough hymen, absence of vagina, very narrow vagina.

Uterus :—Infections, like septic conditions, gonorrhoea or syphilis, etc., tumours and overgrowths; cervix may be tightly closed naturally or after infection and fibrosis; underdeveloped, i.e. infantile uterus.

Fallopian tubes :—The lumen gets blocked due to some chronic infection, like septic conditions—gonorrhoea, syphilis or tuberculosis. On account of a block in the lumen, the ovum cannot travel from the ovaries to the uterus. The block must be bilateral, otherwise the chances of pregnancy are always there.

The potency of the fallopian tubes is tested by means of Rubin's test; i.e., the air is blown inside the uterus to see whether there is any obstruction in the tubes or not.

Ovaries :—In certain cases, the ovaries may be non-functioning by nature or involved in some disease, like tuberculosis, gonorrhoea, syphilis or mumps, or by excessive irradiation.

The operation of dilatation and curettage is done on the uterus and the scrapings are examined under the miscroscope to see the decidual phase of the endometrium, to know the normal functioning of the ductless glands and ovaries in particular and the changes they produce inside the uterus to receive and imbed the fertilized ovum.

This operation serves two purposes.

(i) diagnostic, and

(ii) sometimes curative, when the carvix becomes open (dilated) and the uterus gets fresh growth of endometrium, which may be favourable for the fertilized ovum.

Treatment

1. Examine the husband, his semen for the condition of spermatozoa.
2. Correct the above mentioned causes as far as possible.
3. Improve the general health of the patient. Some people advocate Vitamin E (wheat germ oil) for both husband and wife.
4. Some cases have improved through endocrine therapy, i.e., thyroid and pituitary extracts.
5. In some cases, dilatation and curettage helps.
6. Rubin's test, especially injection of lipoidal into uterus which may open up partial obstruction of the tubes.
7. In very rare cases, major operation of salping-ectomy has to be performed through abdominal opening.
8. Homeopathic remedies :

   Agnus Castus, Borax, Nat. Mur., Selenium, Ac. phos., Calc. Carb., Lyco., Conium, Graph., Medo., Puls., and Sepia.

THERAPEUTIC HINTS

Agnus Castus :—For malesand females both. Premature old age sexually. There is no erection, and the desire is also diminished. In females, there is abhorrence of coitus. Rotten, sad, apprehension of death. Chronic history of venereal disease s often present in males and sexual melancholy in females.

Borax :—This also, fovours easy conception. Dysmenorrhoea of membranous type, worse after menses. Dread of downward motion. Sensitive to noise, sudden noise like that of a gun shot. Frightened, Itching and pruritus vulva.

Conium :—Os is indurated. Usually precancerous stitches in the nipples. Breasts swollen and painful both before and during menses. Ill—effects of suppressed sexual desire as well as of excessive indulgence.

Graphites :—Great anti-psoric remedy. Fat and costive patient. Cracks and blisters. Leucorrhoea white, profuse, excoriating with weakness in the back. Aversion to coitus. Better during and after menses, by warmth and night.

Medorrhinum :—History of suppressed gonorrhoea; it will bring on the discharge. Menses offensive. Blood stain is difficult to wash. Rheumatoid constitution. Os-uteri sensitive. Breasts are sore but cold to touch. Patient is hopeless of recovery. Fear of becoming insane. Fear of dark. Fears someone is following her. Worse sunrise to sunset. Better at night, at seashore; prefers to lie on stomach.

Natrum Mur :—Patient is melancholic, depressed sad and weeping; consolation aggravates Anaemia is marked. Mapped tongue with red insular patches Bearing down pains, worse in the morning; the patient feels as if she must sit down to prevent prolapse. Alongwith these symptoms there is bachache, relieved by lying on the back; throbbing headaches after menses, with soreness of the eyes, especially on turning them. Dryness of vagina. Leucorrhoea is acrid, watery Craving for salt is important.

Thyroidinum :—Patient apparently healthy. The uterus is very small in size. Excessive obesity. Uterine Fibroid, Fibroid-tumours of the breast. Fatigued easily, with weak pulse, tendency to fainting, palpitation, cold hands and feet, low blood pressure, chilliness and sensitive to cold.

Pituitary :—Uterus, breasts and other sexual organs are not fully developed; uterine intertia, the muscular activity is diminished. High blood pressure, vertigo, difficult mental concentration, confusion and fullness deep in frontal region. It also regulates the action of corpus-luteum in sterile women and favours conception in many cases.

Sepia :—There is irregularity of menses with leucorrhoea and constipation; they are too late and scanty or early and profuse, with sharp cutting pains. Violent stitches upward, in the vagina, from uterus to umbilicus. Leucorrhoea is yellow, greenish; with much itching. Prolapse of the uterus and vagina; vagina painful especially on coition. Lack of affection for those whom she loved before is a marked mental symptom.

Lycopodium :—Patient is melancholic and is afraid to be alone; extremely sensitive ; has loss of sell confidence and of memory. Dyspepsia and flatulence. Fullness in stomach after eating a little, with bitter taste in mouth. Incomplete burning eructations rise only to pharynx and there they burn for hours. Liking for warm food and drink. Menses are too late; last too, long, too profuse. Vagina is dry ; so, coition is painful, making conception difficult. Right overy affected, giving pain. Leucorrhoea is acrid, with burning in vagina. The so-called carbo-nitrogenoid constitution. Down with hepatic and kidney affections ;sterility seems to be concerned with them. Premature senility marked.

Selenium :—More indicated in male patients. Loss of sexual power with lascivious fancies. Sexual neuraesthenia. Irritability after coition. Patient has lascivious thoughts with impotency. Gets tired after mental exertion. Extreme sandess.

Acid Phos :—Menses too early and profuse, with pain in liver. Itching; yellow leucorrhoea after menses. Marked debility; mental first, and then physical. Young people who grow rapidly, and who are overtaxed, mentally and physically. Patient is apathetic, and indifferent; listless; impaired memory. Confusion of head is present. In males, the sexual power is deficient; parts relax during embrace. Sycotic excrescences on the genitals.

Pulsatilla :—History of gonorrhoea may be present. Suppressed menses from getting feet wet, nervous debility or cholorosis. They are late, scanty, thick, dark, clotted, changeable and inter-mittent. Leucorrhoea is acrid, burning, creamy. The medtal picture is characteristic. Where the oestrogen activity is disturbed and defective.

Calcarea Carb :—Uterus easily displaced. Uterine polypi. Sterility with copious menses. Breasts tender and swollen before menses. Nymphomania; easy conception. Menses are too early, too profuse and too long with vertigo, toothache and cold, damp feet; the least excitement causes their return. Obese type of patients are amenable to the action of this remedy.

Natrum Carb :—Discharge of means after an embrace in the women and sterility as a result.

Thuja :—Sterility with leucorrhoea. Anaemia may also be present. Hair on the face and legs of women with offensive sweat about the genitals. History of gonorrhoea is often present.

Abroma Augusta :—In tincture from, given during the menses brings on conception in young married women.

Platina :—Sterility in women with excessive sexual desire. It has cured sterility of 12 year's standing.

Aletris Farinosa :—When sterility is due to weakness of the uterus. This remedy tones up the uterus.

Cannabis Indica :—Dysmenorrhoea with sexual desire; sterility. Menses profuse, dark, painful, without clots. Backache during menses. Uterine colic, with great nervous agitation and sleeplessness.

STERILIZATION

Sterilization means rendering one incapable of reproduction. It is effected by means of an operation which is known as VASECTOMY in males and TUBECTOMY OR TUBAL LIGATION in famales.

In the male, the passage of the spermatozoa from the testes through the vas deferens is blocked so that the seminal discharge does not contain any sperm, and thus he is made sterile. In the same way, in the female also, the passage of the ova from the ovaries to the uterus through the fallopian tubes is blocked so that no ovum reaches the uterus and thus the woman is made sterile.

In either case, the underlying idea is to avoid the union of sperm with an ovum. There is effected, of course, no hindrance in the sexual intercourse.

CHAPTER IX

D & C OPERATION

(Dilation and Curettage)

Technique

1. Clear the bowels.
2. Clean the parts.
3. Put under anaesthesia.
4. Insert a speculum and grasp the anterior cervical lip with volsella and pull the cervix out.
5. Pass a sound to estimate the length of the uterus and confirm its position (retroversion, retroflexion).
6. Dilate the cervix with higgers dilators, increasing the size each time.
7. Put the curette and curette the interior of the uterus. Pass it gently upto the fundus, bring it down finally to the cervix.
8. Flush out the cavity with aseptic solution.
9. Dry the uterus.
10. Pass a wick of gauze into the cavity to act as a drain and pack the vagina loosely. This packing can be removed after 12-24 hours.

Indications for Operation

D & C operation is performed for 3 purposes ;

1. Diagnostic,
2. Therapeutic, and
3. Pre-operative.

1. **Diagnostic Purposes** :—We have to resort to this operation for the diagnosis of the following conditions :—

(i) Sterility.

(ii) Cancer of uterus (body).

(iii) Chorionic epithelioma.

(iv) Dysmenorrhoea.

(v) Functional uterine bleeding.

(vi) Gyptomenorrhoea.

(vii) Uterine polypi.

(viii) Endometeriosis.

2. Therapeutic Purposes :— D & C operation is performed as a therapeutic mensure in the following cases:—

(i) Dysemenorrhoea (only dilatation)

(ii) Functional uterine bleeding.

(iii) Mocous polypus.

(iv) Gyptomenorrhoea.

3. Pre-Operative Purposes :—This operation is also undertaken as a pre-operative measure before other operations on the cervix, uterus, etc.

CHAPTER X
DYSPAREUNIA

The term dyspareunia signifies pain during sexual intercourse.

The causes of this condition may be classified as under :

1. Vaginismus :

By this is meant a condition of painful and spasmodic reflex contraction of the muscles surrounding the vaginal orifice during coitus or during digital examination. The levator-animuscles are chiefly at fault. It may be due to mere nervousness and hysteria, hyperaesthesia of the vulva or some local pathological condition, like, vulvitis, vaginitis and urethritis. (They may, however, give rise to dyspareunia directly and without producing vaginismus).

2. **Physical Causes :**

These include mere incompatibility or aversion to coitus when the marriage is unsuitable or nervouseness especially in the newly married women. Dyspareunia from physical causes may persist for months or years after marriage and lead to much domestic unhappiness.

3. Anatomical Causes :

(i) Smallness of vulva and vagina :-- Congenital and due to under-development, or acquired as a result of cicatrical contraction or atrophy of the vagina, or kraurosisvulvae. In the first instance, the obstacle may be rigid hymen.

(ii) **Inflammatory conditions of vulva, vagina or urethra :--** Under this head may be enumerated vulvitis, vaginitis and urethritis ; ulcers, sores and excoriations of the vulva or vagina; kraurosis-vulvae, an inflammatory condition of the hymen or carunculae myrtiformes ; inflamed bartholin glands ; and urethral caruncle.

(iii) More deep seated conditions :--

Such as, metritis, pelvic inflammation and prolapse of the ovaries. The last mentioned cause is a frequent unsuspected cause of dyspreunia : prolapsed ovaries are nearly always hyperaesthetic, and pressure upon them, whether during intercourse or during vaginal examination, gives rise to acute pain.

Treatment

The treatment consists of correcting the underlying condition and the administration of the medicine accroding to the totality of symptoms plus thc constitution.

Some of the leading remedies are :

Berb. V., Staphis., Cactus G., Plumb. Met., Bell., Platina, Arg. Nit., Kreosote, Lyco., Sepia, Ign., Cauloph., Cimicif., and Coffea.

Therapeutic hints

Berberis Vulgaris :--Urinary symptoms are marked, alongwith the genital symptoms. Frequent urination ; urethra burns when not urinating ; pain in thighs and loins on urinating, Nausea before breakfast. Pinching constriction in mons-veneris, vaginismus, contraction and tenderness of vagina; burning and soreness in vagina. Sexual desire is diminished ; with cutting pain during coition. Menses are scanty, gray mucus, with pain in kidneys and chilliness, pain down the thighs. Leucorrhoea, grayish mucus, with painful urinary symptoms. Neuralgia of ovaries and vagina. Wandering, radiating pains. Acts best in fleshy patients with good livers. The patient is listless, apathetic and indifferent.

Staphisaria :-- Parts are very sensitive, so-much-so that as soon as they are touched, there is contraction of these muscles immediately ; worse by sitting down. Irritable bladder in young married women. Leucorrhoea. Prolapse, with sinking in the abdomen ; aching around the hips. Cystocele. A very common and trouble some symptom found in connection with troubles of the genital organs is backache, which is peculiar, in that it is always wores at night, in bed, and in the morning before rising. It has been effectively given in the cure of condylomata, figwarts, or cauliflower-like excrescences of the genitals and perineum.

Cactus Gr. :-Haemorrhage, constrictions as of an iron band, periodicity and spasmodic pains are marked. Constriction in uterine region, ovaries and vaginal muscles. Dysmenorrhoea, pulsating pains in uterus and ovaries Vaginismus. Menses early, dark and pitchlike ; cease on lying down ; with heart symptoms.

Plumbum Met :—Vaginismus, with emaciation. Hardness of mammary glands. Vulva and vagina are hypersensitive, which condition makes the intercourse difficult. Stitches and burning pains in breasts. Menorrhagia with sensation of a string pulling from the abdomen to the back. Disposition to yawn and stretch the limbs.

Belladonna:-- Dryness and heat of vagina, with great sensitiveness, causing pain at coition. Sensitive forcing downwards, as if all the viscera would protrude at genitals ; again there is bar to intercourse. Pain in sacrum and dragging around the loins. Menses are increased; bright red, too early and too profuse. Cutting pain from hip to hip. Menses are hot and offensive. Mastits : pain throbbing, with redness and streaks radiate from the nipple. Breasts feel heavy : are hard and red. Tumours of the breast, with pain worse lying down.

Platina:-- Vaginismus, with parts hypersensitive and tingling sensation internally and externally. Abnormal sexual appetite and melancholia. Oophoritis with strility. Menses are early and profuse, and dark clotted Patient is arrogani and proud ; has superiority complex over others. Hysterical spasms of the parts are there.

Argentum Nitricum :--Great desire for sweets is characteristic of this remedy. Withered up and dried constitution : the so-called carbo nitro genoid constitution. Time passes slowly ; and she wants to do things in a hurry. Trembling in parts felt by the patient. Left ovary is painful ; causes pain during intercourse.

Kreosote :--Corrosive itching withing the vulva, burning and swelling of the labia ; violent itching between labia and thighs. Haemorrhage after intercourse. Burning and soreness in external and internal parts. Intermittent flow of menses. Painful coition due to ulcerations and cancerous affections. Patient does not want to indulge in sexual gratification as she is afraid of bleeding after the act.

Lycopodium :-- Vagina is dry ; pains in the right ovary ; so, the coition is painful. Menses are late ; they last long and are profuse.

Sepia :—Prolapse of the uterus and vagina; parts are relaxed; the pelvis is short ; hence, experiences painful intercourse. Leucorrhoea yellow, greenish ; with much itching.

Caulophyllum :— Extraordinary rigid os. Dysmenorrhoea. Spasmodic and severe pains, which fly in all directions.

Cimicifuga :— Bruised feeling in vagina. Ovarian neuralgia ; pain shoots upward and down the anterior surface of the thighs ; pain across the pelvis, from hip to hip.

Cocculus :— Dysmenorrhoea, with dark profuse menses. Purulent, gushing leucorrhoea between the periods, very exhausting, so much so that she can hardly speak. Especially indicated in light-haired females, with much nausea and backache, unmarried and childless women sensitive and romantic girls.

Coffea :—Dysmenorrhoea, with large clots of black blood. Hypersensitiveness of the vulva and vagina, hence, dyspareunia as a result.

CHAPTER XI

PUBERTY

Puberty means the period marked by the beginning development of secondary sex characteristics.

Usual age of puberty in our country is 12-14 years. The menstruation starts with the onset of puberty. Alongwith the menses, there are certain other changes which take place at this age; e.g.

1. Enlargement of breasts.
2. Enlargement of thyroid gland.
3. Enlargement of parotid glands.
4. Growth of hair on the symphysis pubis and in the axilla.
5. Acnes on the face.
6. Mons veneris, vulva and vagina become fully developed.
7. Body of uterus enlarges and the ratio between the body cervix becames 2 : 1, which was 1 : 2 in childhood.
8. The ovaries increase in breadth and mature the graffian follicles.
9. Some laziness, lassitude and headache are commonly present.

For remedies for the complaints incident to this period, kindly refer to the Chapter "Some Common Remedies."

CHAPTER XII

CLIMACTERIC

This is popularly known as MENOPAUSE.

It implies a group of symktoms characterized by amenorrhoea and vaso-motor disturbances, alongwith other symptoms which occur as a result of the physiological cessation of ovarian activity or after surgical removal of the ovaries.

General Features

1. It occurs usually after the age of about 45 years.
2. There are atrophic changes in ovaries, uterus and external genitals.
3. Mammary tissue atrophies, but is often replaced by fat.
4. Vasomotor disturbances occur; hot flushes of varying intensity and frequency are there, alongwith the variable temperament.
5. Only upper part of the body is affected.
6. Mental derangement sometimes occurs following nervous and dyspetic phenomena.
7. Other more variable symptoms include :—
   (i) Palpitation.
   (ii) Dizziness.
   (iii) Shortness of breath.
   (iv) Headache.
   (v) Fatigue.
   (vi) Anxiety.
   (vii) Irritability.
   viii) Sleepiness.
   (ix) Sleep disturbances.

Mode of Onset

Menopause may occur in any one of the following ways :—

1. **Gradual** :—Periods become less and less with great interval in between, complete menopause being effected in about 8-9 months. This process, being gradual, causes least disturbances.

2. **Sudden** :—Periods suddenly stop and amenorrhoea is at once complete. This usually causes severe menopausal complications.

3. **Intermittent** :—Periods of amenorrhoea following severe bleeding in each case, until permanent amenorrahoea takes place, usually in 6-9 months. This is generally due to weak derangement of ovarian secretions (carcinoma).

Common Remedies :

Amyle., Bell., Bellis., Cactus., Cauloph., China., Con., Glon., Ign., Jabor., Kali C., Kreosote., Lach, Mancinella., Murex., Nux M., Nux Vom., Oophorinum., Plumbum., Puls., Sang., Sepia., Sulphur, Ustilago., Zincum V.

THERAPEUTIC HINTS

Lachesis :—For those who have never been well since menopause. It is given for many climacteric troubles, such as haemorrhoids, haemorrhages, vertigo, burning on the vertex and headaches. For women who are worn out by frequent pregnancies, with sudden stoppage of the menses, trembling pulse, headache, flushings of heat and rush of blood to the heat, cold feet and constriction about the heart.

Cimicifuga :—Sinking feeling at the stomach, pain at the vertex and irritability of disposition. Patient is restless and unhappy, feels sad and grieved. For infra-mammary pains on the left side. Sharp lancinating pains in various parts, either nervous or muscular, if they are connected with uterine disturbances.

Bellis Per :—Patient is very tired, wants to lie down and has backache. Sore, bruised feeling in the pelvic region, Traumatism of the pelvic organs, autotraumatism, expresses the condition for which this remedy is to be given. Intolerance of cold bathing is marked under this remedy.

Pulsatilla :—The mental picture would call for this remedy, whatever be the condition of the patient (pathological or physiological). Mild, gentle and yielding disposition; cries at everything; is sad and desponding; weeps about everything; can hardly give her symptoms on account of weeping. Sandy hair, blue eyes, pale face; and inclined to silent grief with submissiveness. Changeableness of symptoms is very much marked; it is seen in the mental as wall as physical plane. The menses flow, and stop, and flow again. If we find the suppression of flow by getting feet wet, it is the remedy. Leucorrhoea is thick, bland and yellowish green. Here, the digestion is often disturbed; bad taste in the mouth, especially in morning' or nothing tastes good, or no taste at all. Dry mouth with no thirst. Patient feels better in cold, open air and cold applications; while walking and moving about slowly.

Sepia :—A great remedy at the climacteric. Pain in uterus, bearing down, comes from back to abdomen, causing oppression of breathing; crosses her legs to prevent the prostrusion of parts. Flushes of heat with perspiration and faintness. Induration with a painful stiffness in the uter'ine region. Prolapse of the uterus. Lack of affection for her occupation, her house hold work, her family or their comfort, even for those whom she loved best. Yellow saddle across the upper part of cheek and nose, and yellow spots on the face.

Sulphur :—Burning is present everywhere, especially feet; hrs to keep them out of bed to cool them. Redness of orifices, as if pressed full of blood. Weak, faint after hot flushes, followed by sweat, especially at 11 A.M. Averse to bathing; the complaints get worse after bathing. Itching eruptions; scratching is followed by buruing. It is often the terminating remedy, to complete the cure and also to avoid recurrances.

Amyl Nitrosum :—Climacteric headache and flushes of heat, with anxiety and palpitation, flushings followed by sweat at climacteric. Hiccough and yawning.

Belladonna :—Menses increased; bright red, too early and too profuse; hot gushes of blood. Violent throbbling headache, with flushed face and red shoot eyes. Cutting pain, from hip to hip; pain in sacrum. Dryness and heat in the vagina.

Caulophyllum :—Atony of the uterus. Menses and leucorrhoea profuse. Dysmenorrhoea, with pains flying in all directions; spasmodic and severe pains. Extraordinary rigrd os. Needle like pains in the cervix. Rheumatism of the small joins often accompanies.

China :—Menses early; dark clots and abdominal distension. Desire too strong. Debiliating leucorrhoea which is bloody; seems to take the place of the usual menstrual discharge. Painful heaviness in the pelvis. Weakness and debility. Pains in limbs and joints, as if sprained; worse slight touch, but hard pressure relieves; she is verv sensitive, with dread of open air.

Conium :—Induration of the os and cervix. Oophoritis; ovary enlarged, indurated; with lancinating pain. Ill-effects of repressed sexual desire or suppressed menses or from excessive indulgence. Leucorrhoea, after micturition. Dull aching in lumbar and sacral region. Mammae lax ānd shrunken, hard, painful to touch; stitches in nipples; wants to press the breast hard with the hand. Muscular weakness, especially of lower extremities. Perspiration of hands. Putting feet on the chair relieves the pain.

Ignatia :—The hysterical element is prominently present. It is especially adapted to the nervous temperament. Women of sensitive, easily excited nature, dark, mild disposition, quick to perceive and rapid in execution. Effects of grief and worry, much sighing. Exaggeration of the violence of complaints. Sinking feeling in the stomach, relieved by taking a deep breath. Pressure as of a sharp instrument from within outward.

Cactus G :—Construction in uterine region and ovaries. Dysmenorrhoea; pulsating pain in the uterus and ovaries. Menese early, dark, pitch-like; they cease on lying down. Heart symptoms accompany; like dyspepia, palpitation, worse lying on left side, at approach of menses. Low blood pressure.

Glonoine :—A good remedy for climacteric disturbances. Great lassitude, on inclination to work; extreme irritability, easily excited by the slightest oppisition. Menses; delayed, or sudden. Cessation with congestive headache; climacteric flushings; surging of the blood to head and heart; sensation of pulsation throughout the body. Itching all over the body. Pain in left biceps. Drawing pain in the limbs. Backache

Feels better taking brandy. Worse. heat, lying down from 6 A.M. to noon.

Kali Carb :—Sweat, backache weakness; these are three prominent indications for its use. Patient is sensitive to every atmosphoric change, and intolerance of cold weather. Fleshy aged people, with dropsical and paretic tendencies. Patient is very irritable; full of fear and imaginations; never wants to be alone and is never quiet or contented. Menses are early and profuse, or late, pale and scanty, with soreness about the genitals; pains from back pass down the gluteal muscles, with cutting in abdomen. Uterine heamorrhage; constant Oozing after copious flow, with violent backache, feeling better by sitting and pressure. Small of back feels very weak, with stiffness. Early morning aggravation. Worse, after coition and cold weather.

Kreosote :—Another good remedy for ailments associated with climacteric period or occuring after that, corrosive itching within the vulva, burning and swelling of the labia; violent itching between the labia and the thighs. Burning and soreness in external and internal parts. Leucorrhoea, yellow, acrid, of the odour of green corn. Haemorrhage after coition. Dragging backache, extending to genitals and down the thighs. Great debility. Cancerous affections of the genitals are particularly amenable.

Mancinella :—Depressed mental state is characteristic, with exalted sexuality. Silent, sad mood; has wandering thoughts; sudden vanishing of the thought; has fear of becoming insane. Dermatitis, with excessive vesiculation, oozing of sticky serum and formation of crusts. Fungoid growths.

Murex :—This remedy is especially adapted to the nervous, lively and affectionate type of women. Patient is weak and run down. The parts are very sensitive; least touch excites violent sexual desire in her; nymphomania. She is always conscious of her womb. Feeling, as if something was pressing on a sore spot in the pelvis; worse sitting. Pain from right side of the uterus to right or left breast. Sore pain in the uterus. Chronic endometritis, with displacement. Prolapse; enlargement of the uterus, with plevic tenesums and sharp pains, extending towards breasts; aggravated by lying down, must keep legs tightly crossed. Leucorrhoea, green or bloody, alternates with mental symptoms and aching in sacrum. Being tumours in the breasts.

Nux Moschata :—Uterine haemorrhage. Menses too long, dark and thick. Leucorrhoea is muddy and bloody. Suppression, with persistent fainting attacks and irresistible drowsiness. Dryness of the vagina and vulva and the skin; also of all mucous surfaces. Complaints attended by flatulent dyspepsia; abdomen is gre tely distended. Patient has hysterical mood laughing, and crying; is confused, and looks as if in a dream; imagines she has two heads. Bursting headache, which is better by hard pressure. Feels sleepy all the time, is a great keynote.

Nux Vomica :—The patient is very irritable, very sensitive, very chilly; cannot bear noises, odours, light, etc.; the least ailment affects her greatly; reproaches others; and always tries to find fault with others. Menses are always irregular; too early and too long; blood black, with fainting spells. Prolapse of the uterus. Nymphomania. Metrorrhagia. Its peculiar constipation; and disturbed state of digestion. Pain in back, lumbar region.

Oophorinum :—Climacteric disturbances in general; or the sufferings occuring after Oophorectomy Has some action on ovarian cysts also.

Plumbum Met :—Vaginismus, with emaciation and constipation. Induration of mammary glands; stitches and burning pains in them. Vulva and vagina very sensitive. Menorrhagia with sensation of string pulling from abdomen to the back. Has disposition to yawn and stretch her limbs.

Sanguinaria :—Circumscribed redness of the cheeks, flushes of heat, determination of blood to head and chest, burning in palms and soles : i.e., complaints incident to climacteric period. Leucorrhoea foetid, corrosive. Menses offensive and profuse. Soreness of the breasts. Uterine polypi. Itching of the axillae before menses.

Ustilago :—Vicarious menstruation. Ovaries burn, pain and swell. Menorrhagia at climacteric. Oozing of dark blood, clotted, forming black strings. Hypertrophy of the uterus. Bleeding from the cervix very easily.

Zincum V. :—Ovarian neuralgia; pain shoots down the limbs, even to the feet. Sciatica; patient cannot sit still; she must keep the legs in constant motion

CHAPTER XIII

DISORDERS OF MENSTRUATION

AMENORRHOEA

The term amenorrhoea denotes the cessation of menstruation between the age of puberty and menopause ; either temporary or permanent.

(Classification)

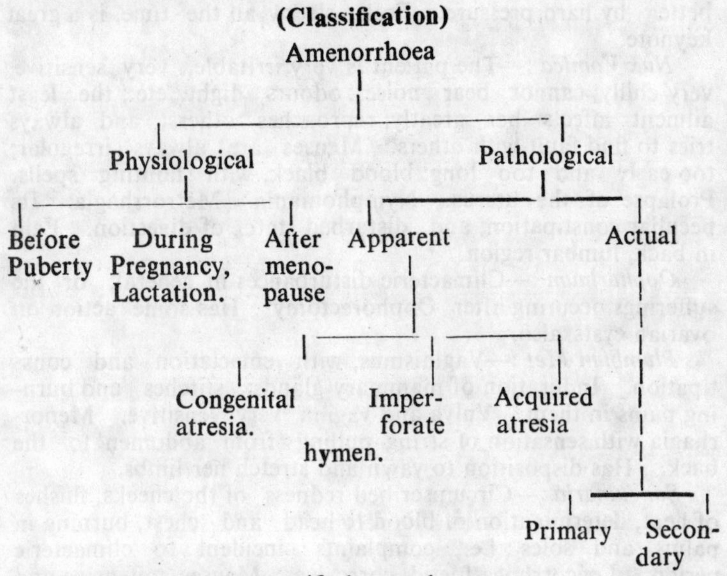

Amenorrhoea may be classified as under :—

1. Physiological.

11. Pathological.

1. Physiological Amenorrhoea :— It may occur in three conditions :—

1. Before puberty, - when the menstruation has not started.

2. During pregnancy and lactation ; and
3. After menopause—when the periods stop.

11. Pathological Amenorrhoea :— Pathological amenorrhoea may be classified into 2 main heads :--

1. Apparent, and
2. Actual.

Apparent Amenorrhoea :-- It is also called **cryptomenorrhoea.** This type of amenorrhoea is said to have taken place when the patient menstruates, but there is no visible discharge. In other words, it is concealed menstruation due to some obstruction in the genital tract.

Causes

(i) Congenital : defects especially imperforation of the lower end of vagina and atresia of cervix, there is no opening in the cervix.

(ii) **Imperforate hymen.**

(iii) **Non canalization of the vagina.**

(iv) **Acquired atresia** - which may be due to the aftereffects of labour, sepsis, operation on the cervix and new growths, like cancer, polypi, etc.

(v) **In duplication of the uterus.** the cavity of one corner may not communicate with the cervix.

Blood accumulates in the vagina -the condition is known as haematocolpos. After some time. the vagina becomes full and the blood starts accumulating in the uterus. (haematocolpometra). Later on. when the uterus is full, the fallopian tubes become full (haematosalpinx) and lastly the condition is known as Pelvic-haematocele.

Clinical Features

(i) Pain in the lower abdomen every month lasting for 3-5 days.

(ii) Persistent heaviness in the lower abdomen.

(iii) Primary amenorrhoea.

(iv) Extreme constipation.

(v) Retention of urine.

(vi) There may be swelling in the lower abdomen with fever (when haemato cells are formed with irritation of the peritoneum).

(vii) Per abdomen, there may be tense cystic swelling in the hypogastric region which may be due to full bladder or due to haematometra and haematocolpos.

(viii) Vaginal examination reveals bluish tense swelling bulging imperforate hymen.

(ix) Per rectum, the vagina feels like tense cystic swelling through the anterior rectal wall.

The treatment consists of drainage of haematocolpos by a crucial incision on the imperforate hymen under general anaesthesia.

Actual Amenorrhoea :-- Actual pathological amenorrhoea is further divided into:--

A. Primary, and

B. Secondary.

Primary Pathological Amenorrhoea :-- This is applied to those cases in which menstrual function is delayed past the usual age of menarche (18 year's age is taken as the upper limit).

Causes

(*a*) *General systemic disturbances* --

(i) Tuberculosis.

(ii) Severe anal infection.

(iii) Anaemia.

(iv) Toxaemia.

(v) Cardiac diseases.

(vi) Hypoproteinaemia.

(*b*) *Pituitary lesions* :--

(i) Tumour formation.

(ii) Inflammation of anterior pituitary gland in childhood disturbs the normal functioning and leads to retardation of growth.

The conditions are due to the absence for deficiency of pituitary hormone.

(iii) Pituitary dwarfism.

1. Short stature.
2. Amenorrhoea.
3. Under developed genital organs, but no lack of secondary sex characters.
4. Forhlich's syndrome.

(c) Diseases of other ductless glands

(i) Cretinsm (hypothyroidism) in childhood and Myoedema (hypothroidism) in adult age.

These are due to the disturbance in the pituitary-ovarian mechanism.

(ii) Adrenal cortex :

Congenital adreno - genital syndrome

The amenorrhoea in this condition is due to the inhibitory effect of adrenogenic hormone on the ovarian function.

(d) Genital lesions.

(i) Ovaries :

(1) Absence of ovaries.

(2) Pelvic inflammatory process such as tuberculosis and peritonitis in childhood may cause destruction of the ovarian tissue.

(ii) Uterus :

(1) Absence of uterus
(2) Uterine hypoplasia
(3) Infantile uterus
(4) Rudimentary uterus
(5) Pubescent uterus.

Functional Amenorrhoea or Hypothalamic Amenorrhoea

This condition is primarily due toga psychosomatic disturbance, which is itself transitory but has a1 profound effect on the endocrinal system

It is estimated that 60% of the cases of amenorrhoea are functional in origin.

Psychological stimuli affect the hypothalamus which depresses the activity of pituitary as a secondary manifestation. The hypothalamic origin is responsible for the obesity which occurs in 50% of cases.

Causes

1. Grief,
2. Worry,
3. Anxiety,
4. Depression,
5. Sexual disharmony,
6. Change of environment, and
7. Change of occupation.

The effect of these factors depends upon the mental status of the individual patient.

Secondary Pathological Amenorrhoea

(a) Uterine causes :

(i) *Developmental* :—(1) Hypoplasia of uterus.

(2) Excessive fibroids of uterine musculature.

(ii) *Injury* :—(1) Hysterectomy (removal of uterus).

(2) Excessive radiation by X-ray or radium, causing destructive changes.

(3) Super-involution ; because the mother continues breast feeding for a long time.

(4) Excessive curettages.

(iii) *Refractory* :—Oestrin and Progesterone cannot produce the necessary changes in the uterine endometrium. Therefore, it is said to be refractile.

TEST :—

Give 5 mgs. of oestrin by mouth for 10 days, then stop. If the bleeding starts within 48 hours, the endometrium is not refractile.

Ovarion causes :

(i) *Developmental* :—Aplastic or hypoplastic ovary is underdeveloped.

TEST :—

Give 10 mgs. of progesterone by mouth for 5 days, then stop. If the bleeding starts within 48 hours, the ovary is not at fault.

(ii) *Injury* :—(1) Oophorectomy.

(2) Radium or X-ray.

(iii) *Tumours* :—Bilateral tumours of the ovaries cause amenorrhoea, but not unilateral in which cases the normal function is carried on by the other ovary.

(iv) *Polycystic ovary in metroplated haemorrhages* :—The patient complains of amenorrhoea for 2/3 months followed by menstruation lasting for 10/15 days or even longer. It is due to the formation of multiple cysts in the ovary.

(v) *Sclerocystic disease of the ovaries* :—Causing fibrosis of the ovaries.

(c) Anterior pituitary causes

(1) Organic diseases

Cushing's syndrome :—It is due to basophilic adenoma of anterior pituitary gland.

Its features are :—

(a) Age : 20-30 years.
(b) Amenorrhoea.
(c) Glycosuria.
(d) Obesity : localised in the face, neck and trunk.
(e) Loss of pubic and axillary hair.
(f) Hirsutism, i.e., abnormal growth of hair.
(g) Genital regression.
(h) Purpura like ecohymosis.

(2) Simmond's disease :—It is due to necrosis of the anterior pituitary. It dates from child birth during which shock and collapse occur.

Its features are :—

(a) Amenorrhoea.

(b) Emaciation, though appetite is good.

(c) Loss of libido.

(d) Indifference to household work, children and husband.

(e) Atrophy of the breasts and genital organs.

(f) Falling of axillary & pubic hair.

(3) Functional disorders of anterior pituitary

(a) *Dystrophia-adiposo-genitalis* :—It occurs due to disturbances in hypothalamus.

(b) *Frohlich's syndrome.*

1. Amenorrhoea.
2. Patient often suffers from sterility.
3. She becomes elderly primigravida
4. Male type of pelvis or flat pelvis.
5. Uterine inertia.
6. Obesity girdle from marked on the abdomen. breasts, hips, buttacks and proximal parts of the extremities.
7. Genital hypoplasia.

(4) Other endocrinal disorders.

(a) *Adernal* :—In addison s disease (Chronic adrenal insufficiency).

Adreno-genital syndrome :—Hyperplasia, adenoma or cancer of adrenal cortex gives rise to this syndrome.

1. It occurs mostly in adult life.
2. Hirsutism.
3. Obesity, buffalo type.
4. Deepening of the voice.
5. Enlargement of clitoris.
6. Regressive changes in the genitals

7. Hypertension.
8. Glycosuria.
9. Osteoporosis.

(b) *Thyroid* :—Amenorrhoea may occur in hypothyroidism (due to deficient secretion of gonadotrophic hormone of anterior pituitary) and hyperthyroidism (due to extreme toxaemia or that oestrin is so rapidly secreted that it has no time to exert its influence over the tissues).

(c) *Pancreas* :—Amenorrhoea is seen associated with diabetes.

(d) *Miscellaneous causes*

(i) *Infectious diseases* :—Amenorrhoea of short duration is frequently found accompanying acute specific fevers.

(ii) *Debilitating diseases* :—

(1) Pulmonary tuberculosis.
(2) Nephrities.
(3) Heart diseases.
(4) Respiratory infections
  (a) Bronchitis.
  (b) Empyema, etc.

1 May arise at any age, but is common during adolescence.
2 Marked loss of appetite.
3 Extreme emaciation.
4 Amenorrhoea.
5. Low blood pressure.
6 Slow pulse rate.
7. Low metabolic rate.
8. Marked uterine hypoplasia.

Treatment

1. General

(i) Exercise.
(ii) Change into warmer climate.
(iii) Diet.

(iv) Treatment of general diseases.

(v) Fresh and open air.

(vi) Iron and folic acid.

2. **Surgical:**—Surgical treatment is required in cases of congenital abnormalities, such as imperforate hymen, atresias, etc, and new growths.

3. **Medicinal :**—Homoepoathic medicines should be selected on the basis of constitution, totality of characteristic symptoms of the patient and the pathological condition as well.

Calc., Carb., Calc. Phos., Puls., Nat. Mur., Sulphur., Silicea, Ferrum Met., Sanguinaria, Graph.: China., Cham., Helon,, Kali Carb., Conium, Opium, Verat. Alb. Coffea, Colocynth. Hyosc., Ign., Staph., Lach., Zinc.. Cocc, Apis, Lil. Tig., Platina.' etc.

Therapeutic hints

Pulsatilia:—This is the first remedy which comes to our mind in cases of amenorrheoa or so--to-say, suppression of menses. Here, the menses flow by fits and starts or when they are suppressed by getting feet wet ; it is also to be thought of when the first menses are delayed in chlorotic girls. Patient is of mild, gentle and yielding nature ; and is easily moved to tears. She is chilly but feels better in the open air : so wants to keep the windows open. Changeability of symytoms (mental as well as physical) is very marked. The pains are of wandering and shifting character.

Calcarea Carb:— Patient is fat, fair and flabby. Here also, the first menses are delayed ; but, there is congestion of head or chest in it. Patient perspires easily about the head and is subject to acidity of the stomach, Palpitation of the heart ; dyspnoea worse ascending and by cold damp feet.

Cimicifuga :-- When the reflex nervous system is disturbed pain in the ovarian regions ; it shoots up and down in the anterior surface of the thighs; across the pelvis from hip to hip. Intolerance of pains, worse morning and cold ; better by warmth and eating. In suppression from a cold, mental emotions and febrile symptoms ; when rheumatic pains in the limbs, or instense headache,or uterine spasms are present,

Ferrum Met :--First menses are delayed, when there is debility, languor, palpitation, sickly complexion and puffiness about the ankles. It responds to weakly. chlorotic women with flushed face, or pale and livid with blue margins about the eyes. It is especially useful in those who have given quinine and nervines.

Sepia i--Insufficient and slow menses in feeble and debilitated Patients, those of derk compiexion, delica'e skin and who are sensitive to all impressions. First menses delayed where leuco rrhoea occurs in stead of menses with congestion of blood to chest and pale face.

Apis :–In young girls, who are constantly busily engaged in this or that, but do nothing right ; who let everything fall out of their hands or break it, and laugh over it ; also great congestion of the head, and even delirium ; oedematous swelling of the lower extremities.

Cocculus :-- Instead of the monthly flow cramps deep in the abdomen ; presure in the chest; dyspnoea ; groaning and moaning ; great weakness, so that the patient is scarcely able to speak ; paralytic feeling in the lower extremities.

Cuprum :-- Typical paroxysms of the most violent cramps in the abdomen, extending up into the chest, with nausea, retching and vomiting ; convulsive motions of the limbs, with piercing shrieks,

Digitalis :-- Age of puberty ; dark red ; bluish colour of the face ; distedned veins on eyes, ears lips and tongue ; constant yawning ; irregular action of the heart ; suffering feeling in bed ; frequent desire to urinate ; leucorrhoea ; painful and swollen feet and limbs, with paralytic feeling in them. Bloody expectoration or nosebleed.

Graphites : -- After Pulsatilla ; congestion of the head and chest ; dark redness of the face ; constriction of the chest ; when lying, with anxiety ; itching between the fingers, and tetters ; nails grow thick and crooked ; the limbs upon which she lies go to sleep.

Kali Carb. :--Age of puberty ; spasms of thee chest ; swlling of the face, especially over the eyes ; stiffness and pain in the small of the back ; dryness of the skin is easily frightened sleepless after 3 o' clock in the morning. feeling worse in all respects at that time. Spitting of blood before the menses ; corroding leucorrhoea ; pain in the anterior part of the thigh.

Lycopodium :- Suppresssion from a fright; great agitation of the blood in the evening, or a feeling as though circulation had ceased ; great desire for sweet things : sour belching ; great fullness in the stomach and bowels ; liver spots on the chest. Headache, sour vomiting, swelling of the feet, fainting fits, and leucorrhoea. When she attains the age of 16, 17 or even 18 without menstrnation ; the breasts do not develop and the ovaries do not perform their function.

Mercurius :-- Cessation of the menses for several months ; headache ; weakness of sight ; nervous trembling of the hands : earthy colour of the face : prolapse uter : diarrhoea with tenesms; oedematous swelling all over; tearing in the limbs, worse at night in bed, with constant sweating.

Natrum Mur. :-- Age of puberty ; melancholy and sadness or hastiness and impatience , awakes with headache ; has frequent fluttering of the heart ; the tongue is covered with small blisters, or shows the appearance of a so-called map-tongue ; the bowels are costive and move with great difficulty, So-called map and there is cutting pain in the urethra after urination.

Phosphorus :-- Menses too late, or dot appearing ; tight feeling in the chest, with dry. tight cough, and spitting of blood, worse before midnight ; bloatedness below the eyes : a great deal of vertigo ; leucorrhoea during the menses.

Senecio gracilis :-- Suppression ; inability to sleep, nervous irritability ; loss of appetite ; coated tongue ; bowels constipated constant feeling of lassitude ; disinclined to move about ; wandering pain in back and shoulders. Is called the female regluator".

Sulphur :-- Great congestion to the pelvic organs and to the head ; cold feet and head on the top of the head ; the patient is very irritable, and inclined to religious reveries , chronic inflammation of the eyelids or other psoric eruptions , dreads to wash with cold water ; feels exhausted from talking ; all worse when standing ; sleepy in the daytime , sleepless at night; great agitation of the blood in the whole body.

——

CHAPTER XIV

DYSMENORRHOEA

Dysmenorrhoea is a condition of painful menstruation where the patient cannot perform her daily work. It is one of the most frequent gynaecological complaints of the young unmarried girls.

Types

A. Congestive.

B. Spasmodic.

C. Membranous.

A. **Congestive Dysmenorrhoea** :—It is also called premenstrual, secondary, extrinsic or acquired dysmenorrhoea.

It course due to pelvic faults. i.e., some lesion in the pelvis. Three main causes have been described by standard books :—

1. Infection.
2. Acquired displacement.
3. Congestion, mostly due to chronic constipation.

1. **Infection** .—Fallopian tube is the most common site of infection to take place, but the ovaries are also involved infection may be :—

(i) Puerperal.

(ii) Post-operative.

(iii) Venereal.

(iv) From bowels, e.g., appendicitis.

(v) Of adhesions of ovarian cysts, etc., to the bowels.

(vi) Through the blood stream, e.g., tuberculosis.

(vii) Through the pelvis, e.g., endometeriosis. salpingitis, salpingoophoritie, pelvic cellulitis, parametritis, etc.

(viii) It is a common symptom of adenomyomata, ovarian cysts, submucous fibroids and polypi.

Dysmenorrhoea is premenstrual unless the uterus is involved, when it is menstrual as well. Here, the pain is of aching and tearing character. This pain is due to the adhesions causing a sense of weight and stretching.

2. **Acquired Displacement** :—It may be due to :

(i) Puerperium.

(ii) Retroflexion.

Here, the fundus of the uterus lying over the veins produces congestion; thereby the endometrium becomes oedematous. The pain is thus premenstrual as well as menstrual often due to oedema of prolapsed ovraies. Prolapse, though rare, is also due to congestion and thus the pain is premenstrual.

3. **Effects of Choronic constipation :**—By toxaemia and loaded pelvic colon obstructing the left ovarian vein which causes congestion and varicosity of the broad ligament and ovaries.

B. Spasmodic Dysmenorrhoea :—It is also known as primary, menstrual, intrinsic or idiopathic dysmenorrhoea.

The actual causation and mechanism is uncertain (as the very name, idiopathic, suggests); but probably it is due to spasmodic contractions of the uterine muscles. The predisposing stimulus to the overactivity of the uterine muscles may be associated with many factors :—

1. **Ill-Development of Uterus :**—The uterus, in cases of severe dysmenorrhoea is generally found to be ill-developed prepubescent or infantile uterus. The size is smaller than the normal uterus after puberty. The cervix may be very slender and thin with a pin hole external os.

2. **Mal-Development of Uterus :**—The uterus may be bicornuate or septate.

3. **Mal-Position of Uterus :**—(i) Uterus may be acutely anteflexed with a fully developed uterus. As it is fully developed, so menstrual pain is not so severe. Here dilatation may be beneficial but the symptoms may recur. Pregnancy again may cure the condition.

(ii) Congenital retroversion.

(iii) Uterus may be displaced laterally to one side.

4. **Defect in Myometrium :**—Underdeveloped musculation of the uterus : There may be preponderance of fibrous tissue ; or plain muscle-fibres are less than normal : with there sult that it lacks in its contractile power so that menstrual blood instead of being forced through the cervix becomes bent up in the body and by distension actually caused produces the pain.

5. **Deficient Polarity :**—Law of Polarity is disturbed ; so there is difficulty in discharging the blood through the cervix.

6. **Abnormalities of Menstrual Discharge :**—Deficiency of thrombolysin or the enzyme secreted by the endometrium during menstruation puts to liquidise the menstrual clots in the uterus : when these clots are discharged. the pain is experienced.

C. **Membranous Dysmneorrhoea :**—It is due to the exfoliation of membranes of the uterus. The exfoliation may be deep or superfical giving rise to thick or thin clot. The clots are very rarely complete and come out in half or smaller pieces. The cause of this is yet unknown but it is thought to be due to some upset in the endocrine control of the uterus. Sometimes thin casts as well as thick casts are often passed without pain ; but when retained for sometime, they become rolled up with blood to form as solid casts and then the dysmenorrhoea is severe. The patients are usually sterile, but it may occur in parous women also. Here pregnancy makes the condition worse.

Its treatment is as follows :—

(i) Improve the general health of the patient.

(ii) Sex abstinence.

(iii) Curetting cures a few cases.

(iv) When menorrhagia is present, treat the patient with Sabina, Calc. Carb. or any other indicated remedy.

(v) X-ray and radium treatment is often recommended alongwith hysterectomy also in incurable cases.

Clinical Features and Symptoms

Congestive Dysmenorrhoea :—

1. Pain starts 3-4 days before menstruation.
2. Dull aching pain which is not so severe.

3 Pain is worse by discharges.

4. Profuse blood

5 On P.V. examination, signs of pelvic inflammation are detected. Congestive dysmenorrhoea usually occurs a few years after painless menstruation.

6. Feeling of weight and heaviness in the lower abdomen.

Spasmodic Dysmenorrhoea :–

1. Severe excruciating pain which is intermittent and spasmodic in nature.
2. Pain is felt in the lower abdomen and often down the thighs.
3. Pain starts usually on the first day of the menses which may last either for the first few hours or may continue throughout the period, the intensity becoming less severe.
4. Pain is not better by the discharge.
5. Faintness collapse, vomiting or nausea accompanies the pain.
6. On P.V. examination, the following facts are discovered :–
   (i) Ill–developed uterus.
   (ii) Mal–developed uterus.
   (iii) Mal–position of the uterus
7. The menstrual cycle is a little irregular and the amount of blood lost during each period is less than the average.

Membranous Dysmenorrhoea

1. Severe excruciating pain with faintness, collapse with the onset of menses.
2. With the spasm of pain, the membrane (uterine cast) is shed off.

In typical cases, spasmodic dysmenorrhoea arises at puberty. It is rare to see cases of severe spasmodic dysmenorrhoea in women over the age of 35 years. Patients who are sterile do not usually give a history of spasmodic dysmenorrhoea.

Diagnosis :

Diagnosis is confirmed by signs and symptoms and physical examination.

Treatment

1. **General** :—General treatment is of great importance.

(i) Open air exercise, no sedentary habits.
(ii) Avoid constipation.
(iii) Treat other general diseases.
(iv) Liquid and nourishing diet.
(v) Sometimes dysmenorrhoea is rendered by marriage and child birth. So, those cases are to be dealt with accordingly, such as psychologically, etc.

2 **Surgical**

(i) D & C operation.
(ii) Px. sacral sympathectomy.
(iii) Hysterectomy.
(iv) Plastic surgery if cervix is not developed.

3. **Hormonal** :—Oestrin may be given to help regulate the hormonal activity of the ovaries, so as to inhibit ovulation causing painless menstruation. It is given immediately after cessation of menses for one week (5 mg. t.d.s.).

Progesterone inhibits uterine contractions. It may be given before the onset of menstruation (2-3 mg. daily for 3 days).

4. **Accessory** :—Measures to relieve pain; such as hot applications on the abdomen and rest during periods.

5. **Medicinal**

(a) Congestive dysmenorrhoea

Aco., Arn,, Bell., Puls., Sabina, Sepia., Lach., Zinc.

(b) Spasmodic dysmenorrhoea

Cham., Actea racemosa, Cauloph., Kali Phos., Melilotus, Pendulum, Xanthoxylum, Verat. Vir.

(c) Membranous dysmenorrhoea

Borax, Ustilago, Viburnum opulus.

(d) Constitutional remedies.

Calc. Carb., Nat. Mur., Sepia, Lyco., Sulphur, Nux Vom., etc.

Limitations of Homoeopathic Treatment

As far as the condition is only functional or slightly pathological, it can be treated and set right with the medicines. But, if the condition (i.e. dysmanorrhoea) is attributed to mal and ill-developmental of the uterus or to some other congenital defect of the genital organs, or if marked with gross pathological changes, e.g., adhesions, it cannot be treated with medicines alone. In such cases, mechanical interference is of prime importance. Apart from these measures, hormonal treatment is also required in some cases. If all this is correct, i.e., the obstacles to cure are removed, the rightly selected medicine will bring about very good and satisfactory results.

THERAPEUTIC HINTS

Congestive dysmenorrhoea

Aconite :—Dysmenorrhoea from thickening of the peritoneum over the ovaries. Congestive type, with violent headache; labour-like pressing in the uterus; restlessness; necessity to bend double on account of pain but finds no relief in any position; tossing about.

Apis :—Violent labour-like, bearing-down pains, followed by discharge of scanty, dark, bloody mucus; stinging pain in the ovaries; scanty, dark urine; wax coloured skin.

Arnica :—Pain with extreme tenderness in the lower abdomen; fear of being touched. Having a history of fall.

Belladonna :—Congestive enlargement of the uterus of the ovaries, especially right ovary. Bearing down pain, as if the contents would be expelled out. Discharge bright red, hot, offensive clots, blood thick. Pain comes and goes suddenly. Pain worse walking, sitting bent; better standing or sitting erect.

Pulsatilla :—The menses are dark in colour delayed; the flow will be fitful and the more severe the pains are the more chilly the petient will get. Wetting of the feet is usually the cause. It has a pain as if sharp stones were rubbing against each other in the abdomen and distension of the abdomen from accumulation of flatus; the pains are worse at night, awaken the patient and make her irritable.

Sabina :—Blood partly fluid and partly clotted. Severe pain from the sacrum to the pubis and vice versa. Red blood with blackish clots. Bleeding worse slightest motion.

Lachesis :—Pain, better when menses starts. Discharge is blackish, acrid and offensive. Genitals sensitive; cannot bear weight of the clothes. Menses too short, feeble and late. Left ovary very painful and swollen, indurated. Mammae inflamed, bluish. Coccyx and sacrum pain, especially on rising from sitting posture.

Zincum :—Dysmenorrhoea with mamia. Fidgety feet. Pain in left ovary, better at the onset on flow.

Lapis albus :—Pain is also severe that she would fall unconscious; relief at the flow starts. Dark clots and black lumps of blood on first day. Likes to be out of doors.

Spasmodic Dysmenorrhoea

Chamomilla :—Suitable to nervous, irritable patients. Severe labour like, colicky and tearing pains; pains drawing from small of back to the front, down the things. Griping and pricking in uterus followed by a passage of large clot. Flow often starts in ebbs; abundant when it comes. Snappish during discharge of profuse clotted blood. Dark, clotted blood.

Cimicifuga :—Rheumatic dysmenorrhoea. Rheumatic pains during menses (bigger joints). Blood is blackish, partly fluid and partly clotted. Shooting pain in the abdomen radiating from one side to another; also labour like. Great debility after and between the periods. The more the flow the more the pain.

Caulophyllum :—Spasmodic irregular and very severe pains, especially the first two days of the menses. Intermittent pains in the groins, broad ligaments or even chest and limbs. Sympathetic cramps in the bladder and rectum. Pain in small of back and great aching soreness in lower limbs. (Pains from retroversion or a relaxed flabby condition of the uterus).

Kali Phos :--Uterine pains after alternating with severe night drain. Pains worse pressure. Nervous exhaustion and feeling of faintness. Too late, too profuse menses with thin deep red blood.

Melilotus :—Menses painful, difficult, with congestive headache. Sharp shooting pains in external genitals only for a moment, but recurring.

Trillium : – Gushing of bright red blood from the uterus on least movement. Pain in the hips and back as if it were falling to pieces with desire to bind them tightly.

Viburnum Opulus :—Spasmodic and memberanous dysmenorrhoea. Menses late, scanty, lasting a few hours, offensive Crampy pains from back to loins, extending to the thigs. Severe bearing down, aching in sacrum and pubic region, excruciating crampy, colicky pains in hypogastrium, much nerveousness and occasional shooting pains in the ovaries; ovarian regions heavy and tender. Pains going around the pelvis and also the empty gone feeling in the stomach.

X*anthoxylum* :—It is useful where the pains are agonizing, burning starting in the iliac regions and extending down the thighs long the crural nerves with a feeling as if the limbs were paralysed, the menses are usally profuse, and with it agonizing bearing down pains; ovarian neuralgia, cheifly left sided. Headache over the left eyes the day before the menses. The patient are of spare habits and of a delicate nervous temperament. She chief characteristic of this remedy is that the patient gets no relief in any position.

Veratrum Viride :--Terrible dysmenorrhoea for several days before the onset of menses, with face and head congested. Tongue white or yellow with red streak down the centre.

Magnesia Phos :--Neuralgic and crampy pains before the flow, better from warmth and pressure and aggravation from motion.

Cocculus :--Profuse discharge of clotted blood and severe headche accompanied by nausea. Uterine cramps with suppressed irregular menses and a sero-purulent bloody discharge.

Colocynth :--Agonizing pain great restlessness, must bend double to find relief. Burning pain in ovary. The pains are better by hard pressure and heat. Women with copious menses, and of sadentary habits. Round small cystic tumours in ovaries or broad ligaments. The patient wants her abdomen to be supported by pressure. Bearing down cramps, causing her to bend double. Patient is extremely irritable; becomes angry when questioned.

Membranous Dysmenorrhoea

Borax :--Menses too early, too profuse, with colic and nausea and pain in stomach extending into small of back. Pruritus of vulva and eczema; aphthae. Dysmenorrhoea with sterility; favours easy conception. Sensation of distension in clitoris with sticking. Leucorrhoea, like white of egg, with sensation as if warm water was flowing. Patient is nervous, sensitive to noise and has dread of downward motion.

Magnesia Phos :--Symptoms already given.

Viburnum Opulus :--Symptoms already discussed.

Ustilago :--Discharge of blood from the slightest provocation. Bright red, and partly clotted blood. Atony and flabby condition of the uterus. Ovaries burn. Profuse menses after miscarriage.

CONSTITUTIONAL REMEDIES :

Calcarea Carb, Calcarea Phos. Sepia. Natrum Mur., Nux Vomica, Sulphar, Phosphorus and Lycopodicum.

Calcarea Carb :--Various complaints, toothache after the menses; nervous debility; pale bloatedness of the face; cannot bear anything tight around the waits; stiffness of the nape of the neck; pain in the back; cold hands and feet; sensitiveness of cold air; bad consequences from washing; scrofulous individuals.

Calcarea Phos :--When during puberty the patient has not been careful, and dysmenorrhoea has resulted from these causes. (J.T. Kent).

Sepia :--Colicky pains and scanty discharge; great bearing down, which obliges her to cross the limbs; morning sickness and great sensitiveness against any smell from cooking; toothache; halfsided headache; nausea; constipation.

Natrum Mur :--Menses scanty and dark; preceded by frontal headaches; often subject to fever-blisters on libs, and during summer to urticarious eruptions. (R.E. Bilding).

Nux Vomica :—Twisting pains moving about in the abdomen, with sickness of the stomach; crampy and stitching pains in the pelvic region; soreness the pubis; cramps in the bladder; constant, unsuccessful urging to defaecate ; after all sorts of drugs and so-called pain-killers.

Sulphur :—Scanty menses of a thick, acrid blood; cramp ; colic; terrible neuralgic pains in the face; much concered about her salvation; congestion to the head and heat on the top of it; spotted redness of the face; cold feet; standing increases the pains; Chornic eruptions here and there.

Phosphorus :—Colicky pains; great fermentation in the bowels; a great deal of vertigo; chronic looseness of the bowels; or chronic constipation, with dry, narrow faeces; slender-built women.

Lycopodium :—Partly black clotted, partly bright red blood, and partly bloody serum, with labour-like pain, followed by swooning; distension of the abdomen in different places, changing localities; pain in the small of back, extending into the thigh ; worse in the afternoon from 4 O'clock, commencing with chilliness; restless sleep; dreams of falling down from a height; especially for women who habitually menstruate profusely.

——

CHAPTER XV

MENORRHAGIA

MENORRHAGIA means an excessive menstrual flow. It can be divided into 3 main groups according to the age :--

1. Menorrhagia at puberty.
2. Menorrhagia at child bearing age.
3. Menorrhagia at menopause.

1. Menorrhagia of Puberty

It coincides with the onset of menses. The bleeding may be continuous or it may be with short intervals in between or it may be protracted or prologed type of period lasting for days.

Aetiology :

In the great majority of cases, the underlying cause is pituitary or ovarian dysfunction similar to that occuring in the later life, i. e., at menopause. There may be hyperthy. roidism or sometimes hyperfunction of the thyroid gland with deficiency of calcium in the blood.

In allopathy, calcium lactatel is prescribed with para-thyroid alkaloids and anterior-pituitary preparations, like Prolan, etc. They also sometimes recommend deep X-rays and irradiation, but when applied to the pelvis it causes perma-nent amenorrhoea. In some cases, curettage is also done.

2. Menorrhagia at Child bearing age

The causes of this menorrhagia may be classed under two haeds :—

A. General and

B. Local.

A. General Causes

(i) Blood diseases ; e.g., pern'cious anaemia, purpura or scurvy.

(ii) Chronic nephritis, because it raises the blood pressure.

(iii) Nervous diseases ; e.g , mania.

(iv) Use of alcohol.

(v) Hot climate.

(vi) Endocrinal factors ; too ferquent ovulation resulting in shortening of the menstrual cycle (epimenorrhoea - short cycle of periods).

B. Local Clauses

(i) Infection of the uterus, tubes, ovaries and pelvic peritoneum.

(ii) Chronic metritis, including chronic sub-involution.

(iii) Metropathia-haemorrhagica : it is a condition in which the uterus is likely to bleed excessively.

(iv) New growths in the uterus ; e. g., fibroids, adenoids, etc.

(v) New-growths of the ovaries, tubes, and retention cysts of the ovaries.

(vi) Displacement of the genital organs especially the uterus ; e.g., retroversion cum prolapse causing endometritis.

Me norrhogia of Menopause

Aetiology

(i) Hyperthyroidism after cessation of ovarian secretions ; such patients are usually very irritable and may have tremors.

The allopaths follow the treatment as under :--

(a) Rest in bed.

(b) Calcium lactate , and

(c) Pituitary extracts.

(ii) Unequal ovarion activity : This may cause irregular menorrhagia owing to the atrophying ovaries which do not produce much secretions to bring on the menses at the proper time. When enough secretion is produced, profuse and protracted bleeding occurs.

(iii) Teumours : Cancer is most important, because the woman is more than 45 years of age.

(iv) Fibrosis of muscular wall of the uterus and of its blood vessels : they become hard and thus crack.

(v) Fibrosis of the endomenstrium due to old age. Here all the menstrual blood does not escape owing to the density of fibrosis and, therefore, small collections of blood are scattered here and there under the endometrium. This acts as a foreign body and nature wants to throw it out in menorrhagia and so menorrhagia occurs. Here, again, some cases are helped by curettage.

Treatment

General

1. Rest in bed.
2. In severe cases, curettage has to be resorted to.
3. X-ray or irradiation should not be allowed.
4. Removal of the underlying cause, as far as possible.
5. Liquid nourshing diet.

B. Hormonal

Oestrin and Progesterone preparations.

6. Medicinal

Aletris Farinosa, Ammon. Carb., Aranea, Arn, Ars., Bell., Borax., Cactus, Calc. Carb, Can. Ind., Canth., Cham., China, Cinnamonium, Collinsonia, Croccus, Cyclamen Frig, Ferrum Phos., Geranium, Hama., Helonias, Kali C., Kali Mur., Kreosote, Milles., Nit. ac., Nux V. Phos., Platina Plumb., Sab., Sec., Sepia, Stannum, Trilluim, Xanthoxyllum.

THERAPEUTIC HINTS

Calcarea carb. --Menses too early, too profuse and lasting too long. Cutting pains. Patient is chilly, fat, fair and flabby. Desire for indigestible things, like chalk, earth, charcoal, etc., Anaemic symptoms and congestion of the head and chest; leucorrhoea after the menses; scrofulous diathesis.

Sabina :-- Profuse bright blood. Sexual excitement. History of abortion or threatened abortion. Pain from sacrum to pubic and below upwards in vagina, worse least motion ; feels better in the open air.

Platina:–Dark, clotted blood, with tingling and hypersensitivenees of the parts. Self exaltation, haughty, finds faults with others. Better by walking.

Nymphomania

Bryonia :—Vicarious haemorrhages. Amenorrhoea alternates with menorrhagia. Blood is dark red and profuse, worse least motion. Constipation. Splitting headache, worse on moving the eyes ; white coated tongue ; great thirst ; bilious vomiting ; tearing in the limbs.

Phosphorus :—Bleeding profuse, early and lasting for a long time ; or too late, but very copious ; afterwards great weakness blue rings around the eyes ; loss of flesh and great fearfulness Tall and slender patient with blue eyes ; tender, sensitive women, with frequent heat in the back, and cold legs. She will spit blood during menses.

Secale Cor :—Profuse bleeding of black colour with icy cold extremities in lean and slender women who always suffer from heat. The patient wants to uncover and to be cool. Blood is thin and offensive. There may also be clots in the blood. Spitting of blood before the menses. Leucorrhoea three days after menses.

Ipecac :—Bleeding with prostration. Thin, bright red blod gushes in a stream running through clothes, bed and collecting a pool on the floor. The blood does not coagulate easily. The patient is pale, neuseated and fainting. Blue rings below the eyes.

Belladonna :—Pressure and profuse bleeding with sensation as if everything would fall through the vegina. Foul smelling coagulated blood. Throbbing headache and flushed face.

Stramonium :—With loquacity. Discharge of profuse dark coagulated blood, with drawing pains in the abdomen and thigs.

Ferrum Met :—Early and profuse menses, last long, and causing much debility; with a fiery—red face, whilst at other times the face is pale and earthy looking.

Cocculus :—Menses early and long with prostration; when rising upon the feet, gush out in a stream; paralytic feeling of the lower extremities.

Vinca Minor :—Profuse menses or passive menorrhagia, when the blood flows in a continuous stream ; with debility.

Chamomilla :—Profuse discharge of dark, almost black, coagulated blood with violent, severe, intolerable and maddening pains, from the small of the back to the os pubis; irritable; fainting spells; cold extremities.

China :—Excessive bleeding of long duration, resulting in much debilitated condition; accompanied by flalutent distension of the abdomen. Serves as a tonic in such cases.

Arnica :—Bleeding with a history of injury, fall or below; after mechanical interference at abortion; a very good remedy after labour. With sore, bruised feeling about the genitals and all over.

Nux Vomica :—Menses profuse and too early; highly sensitive patient cannot bear light or noise, is put out of patience when spoken to, gets angry and violent, without any provocation, is head-strong and self-willed, or gets flrightened easily and is almost beside herself from the least thing that may happen; she dreads the fresh air. After coffee, liquors, highly seasoned food, drugs, sedentary life.

Trillium :—Menses every fourteen days, lasting seven and eight days; in between profuse leucorrhoea of a yellowish colour and creamy consistence. The blood is at first bright red, but owing to anaemia, grows pale.

Calcarea Phos :—Menses every two weeks, black and clotted; griping and rumbling in the abdomen before menses; leucorrhoea; stitching pains in the left side of the head; sleepiness during the day.

Ammon Carb :—Premature and very copious flow, especially at night, when sitting or riding and after a ride in the cold air; with spasmodic pains in the belly and hard stools with tenesmus; cholera-like symptoms at the start of the flow.

Cimicifuga:—Menses profuse and too early; dark, coagulated blood; aching in the limbs; severe pain the in back, down the thigs, and through the hibs, with heavy pressing down; weeping wood; nervousness, hysteric spasms; great pain in the head and eyeballs, increased by the slightest movement of the the head and eyeballs.

Coccus cacti :—Flow only in the evenıng after lying down, not when moving about; urging to urinate, but, cannot pass urine until a clot of blood is discharged; attended by nausea and vomiting.

Sepia :—Menses too early or at right time; venous congestion of the head; one sided headache, with nausea and vomiting; loathing of all food; pot-belliedness after confinement; constipation; yellow spots on the face.

Kreosote :—Menses profuse and last too long; great distension of the abdomen before the menses, so that she appears as though she was pregnant; blood offensive; leucrrehoea between the periods; headache before menses; she very obstinate and irritable. Worse on lying down, better from walking about.

Apart from these remedies, all the snake poisons are very effective remedies in such cases.

——

CHAPTER XVI

METRORRHAGIA

METORRHAGIA :—Is the bleeding from the uterus not connected with the periods.

Aetiology

It may be due to the following causes :—

1. Abortion : threatened, inevitable or incomplete.
2. Ectopic gestation.
3. Tumours of the uterus :
   - (i) Sub-mucous polypi or fibroids.
   - (ii) Mucous polypi.
   - (iii) Carcinoma of cervix or body of the uterus.
   - (iv) Chorionic epithelioma.
   - (v) Sarcoma of uterus, though rare.
4. Nephritis ard high blood pressure.
5. Acute pyosalpinx in some cases.
6. Torsion of the pedicles of ovarian cyst, in certain cases.

If none of these causes is found, it is essential that the patient should be examined under anaesthesia and the uterus is curetted so as to make sure that there is no malignancy. But in some cases, curettage besides being diagnstic may also prove curative by removing a polypus or in infected pouch in the endometrium.

Treatment

Treatment is almost the same as under menorrhagia: i.e.

A, General

(i) Remove the cause, if detected, and as far as possible.

(ii) Rest in bed.
(iii) Liquid and nourishing diet.
(iv) X-ray and irradiation.
(v) Dilatation and curettage.
(vi) Hysterectomy, if malignancy is found.

B. Hormonal

Progesterone and Oestrin.

C. Medicinal

Ambra, Gr., Arnica, Arsenic, Bell., Bovista, Cactus, Calc. Carb., Cauloph., Cham., China, Cinnanonium, Croc., Ferrum phos. Hama, Ipeac, Lach, Nit Acid, Phos, Pyrogen, Rhus Aromatica, Sabina, Secale, Sepia, Stram., Thlaspi, Trillium, Vinaca Minor.

THERAPEUTIC HINTS

Aletris Farinosa :—Menses profuse and premature due to atonic condition of the uterus, with labour—like pains, debility from loss of fluids and sterility. Habitual abortions. Uterine haemorrhages, after abortion or in connection with menses; large clots followed by copious bleeding. Digust for food, nausea and indigestion.

Hamamelis :—Very useful after operation and when the bleeding occurs midway between the periods. Blood is dark, profuse and the abdomen feels sore; worse warm; moist air.

Thlaspi bursa :—Useful in the bleedings of fibroids. Given for the expulsion of clots. Violent uterine colic. Too frequent periods; bleeding and pain is worse, every alternate period. Uterus is very sore on rising early in the morning. Bruised feeling inside the pelvis.

Trillium :—General haemorrhagic remedy. Feels as if hips and back were falling to pieces, better by tight bandaging. Useful in metrorrhagia of climacteric. Faintness and dizziness. Big fibroid cases ; gushing of bright blood on least motion. Relaxation of pelvic region; prolapse, with great bearing down. Crampy pains. Leucorrhoea copious, yellow, stringy.

Carbo Veg :—Menses too early, too long and copious. Prostration with every menstrual flow. Burning in vagina, as if burning coals are but in it. Sensation of emptiness, whenever she puts her child to the breast.

Sabina :—Blood bright red or dark, also in clots, sometimes alternating, now dark, coagulated and then, again thin and bright red ; flows mostly in paroxysms, which are brought on by the slightest motion or it ceases when walking about ; drawing; cutting, pressing pains from the small of the back to the genitals and into the thighs ; women who menstruate early and almost always profusely; gouty diathesis ; when the patient feels better in cool and worse in warm temperatures ; threatening abortion; after miscarriage and confinement.

Belladonna :—Great bearing down as if everything would be pressed out, or a pain from the sacrum through the pelvis to the pubis; the blood feels hot; headache: loss of consciousness, darkness before the eyes ; enlarged pubis ; cold nose ; oppression, groaning, yawning, jerkings of the arms ; convulsive clenching of the thumbs.

Secale Cor :-- Atonic haemorrhages during the critical age; after confinement; dark, seldom coagulating blood, sometimes foetid; no pain, or only slight bearing down; or dreadful bearing-down and dragging-out feeling; flooding, worse from the slightest motion ; trembling, convulsive jerkings of the limbs; cramps in the calves of the legs; general coldness.

Kali Carb :-- Threatening abortion and consequences of it; great weakness in the small of the back and lower extremities; pain in the small of the back as though it were broken; dry, hacking cough; obstinate sweating, with feverish chilliness; chronic inflammatory states of the womb, with nausea and vomiting.

Phosphorus :-- Between the menses and during pregnancy ; lame and bruised feeling in the small of the back; dry cough and tightness in the chest, worse before midnight; great heat on the top of the head or in the spine; a great deal of vertigo, chronic looseness of the bowels, worse in the morning, or else chornic constipation with dry, narrow stools.

Plumbum :--During the climacteric period; dark clots, alternating with fluid blood or bloody serum, with a sensation of fullness in the pelvis and slight bearing—down pains from the small of the back to the front; skin dry, pale, yellowish, here and there "liver spots" great debility, short breath on going up stairs; depressed spiries. Poisoning with lead brings on abortion.

Pulsatilla :-- Dark. coagulated blood emitted in paroxysms; worse in the evening, with labor—like pains; habitual looseness of the bowels, ordinarily rather scanty menses; yielding disposition.

Sepia :—Climacteric age, or during pregnancy, especially during the fifth and seventh months; congestion of the head. fullness and pressure in the chest; spasmodic contractions in the abdomen. with terrible bearing down. induration of the womb: varicose veins yellow, sallow complexion. Such patients are very irritable, and faint from any little exertion.

Sulpher :—In chronic cases, when other remedies do not prevent its return. psoric taint of the system. eruptions here and there, or previously suppressed eruptions; looseness of the bowels early in the morning, or else great constipation. fits of gnawing hunger before dinner; the patient complains of great heat, or flushes of heat; has sleepless nights, seemingly without cause, or on account of a tormenting itching all over the body ; itching about the anus and genitals; chronic leucorrhoea, etc.

Rhus Tox :—Bright red blood: threatening abortion, induced by straining or lifting; trembling sensation in the middle of the chest; contractive pain around the hypochondria; drawing, tearing in the back, loins and hips; cramp-like contraction of the thighs; aching all over, worse during rest; heavy, unrefershing sleep, full of dreams.

Crocus :—Dark, viscid, stringy blood, in black clots; feeling as if something alive were in the abdomen; nervous excitement; palpition of the heart; fearfullness; after being overheated, straining and lifting; after abortion and delivery; worse from slightest motion; yellowish, earthy colour of the face.

Caulophyllum :—Threatening abortion, and with spasmodic bearing—down pains : great vascular excitement ; passive haemorrhage after abortion or confinement; tremulous weakness of the whole system.

Calcarea Carb :—Climacteric period; choronic metrorrhagia. mixed with leucorrhoea; previously always inclined to profuse and protracted menses.

Nux Vomica :—During the climacteric period, and especially if such persons have been drugged previously by allopathic ways, or have used much coffee or alcoholic drinks, or too highly seasoned food ; if they lead a sedentary life, complain much of costiveness and headache, suffer with piles, etc.

Ferrum met :—Partly fluid and partly black, clotted blood ; labour-like headache and dizziness ; constipation and hot urine.

CHAPTER -

LEUCORRHOEA

Leucorrhoea is a very old term meaning literally a white discharge from the vagina, which should only mean a non-purulent discharge and hence should not be used for ineffective type of discharges. But, in fact, the term leucorrhoea has been used to denote all typs of discharges from the vagina, whether ineffective or non-infective, physiological or pathological. Let us take this term in a wider sense, meaning thereby "an abnormal discharge from the vagina."

Leucorrhoea is, as a matter of fact, not a disease but a symptom only. There is hardly any gynaecological condition which does not have this symptom being present.

It is important to know that in health also, there is a certain amount of discharge present in the vagina. The chief source of this secretion is the cervical glands that pour out a glairy moucoid secretion which is definitely alkaline in reaction with a PH value of 7.5 to 7.8. This secretion provides a natural defensive barrier against the ascending infection, because this mucous secretion contains a bacteriocidal action.

Further, this secretion gets mixed up with the vaginal secretion which consists of a transudation alongwith a certain amount of desqumated cells of the vaginal epithelium gives it a lightly cramish white appearance. This secretion is acidic in reaction with a P H value of 4.5 to 5. The acidic reaction is due to the presence of lactic acid produced by the action of Doderlein's bacillus (a non pathogenic bacteria peresent in the vaginal flora) on the glycogen which is deposited in the vaginal epithelium under the influence of oestrin. In adult age, there fore, the vagina is defended against infection by this acidic fluid which is dettimental to the growth of bacteria, especially the pryogenic ones.

Menstruation after delivery or abortion are the occasions when this acidity is partly or whole neutralized by the alkaline blood and hence the infection is more likely to occur at this time. This defensive mechanism is also lacking in children on account of absence of oestrin and hence they are more prone if exposed to infection, e g., bathing in contaminated water, playing in dit or debilitated by other diseases. In the port-menopausal period also the women are again prove to infection an account of diminsihed oestrin which is associated with atrophic changes in the genital tract accompanied with diminished blood supply to these organs.

Aetiology

As leucorrhoea is a symptom of vorious gynaecological conditions, physiological as well as pathological, it is important to understand that the underlying factor in most of these conditions is congestion of the pelvic organs which inevitably results in an increased activity of the cervical, endometrial and vaginal epithelium to produce an excessive secretion. This excessive discharge may be physiological, or pathalogical infective or non-infectiae:--

1. The most common conditions, in which excess of this discharge is likely to be present are pregnancy, premenstrual or menstrual periods, ydrorrhoea gravidarum and congestion of the uterus.
2. Irritation due to mechanical factors, e.g., use of chemical contraceptives, pessaries, intrauterine devices, etc,, may also establish chronic inflammatory process causing congestion and hence leucorrhoea.
3. Pathological conditions of the female genital.organs, e.g., infection, growths and displacements, etc., also produce the same phenomenon, i.e., congestion and leucorrhoea.
4. Recently, endocrinal factors have been given a great deal of prominence as a possible cause of leucorrhoea as is clear by the fact that the non-infective erosion is due to excess of oestrin in the system. Pregnancy and menstrual periods are also examples of hyper-secretion due to large amounts of oestrin in the blood at those periods.
5. Psychogenic causes, e.g., worries, anxiety, overwork, and sexual excitement without fulfilment may also cause chronic

leucorrhoea. It may seem strange, though it is now certain that emotional upsets affect hypothalamus, which in turn upsets the gonadotrophic functions of the pituitary gland, so much so that even anovulation has been caused by mental stress and emotional situations. Considering the close relationship between pituitary, ovarian functions, glncogen deposition and PH value of vaginal-flora, the hormonal theory also seems to be a possible cause.

6. Errors in diet, excessive use of stimulants, e. g., tea, coffee, alcohol, smoking, all these things have been suggested to cause leucorrhoea it seems to be possible because of the absorption of toxic substances or by stimulating the nervous mechanism of gland causing hormonal imbalance. It is also suggested that faulty and deficient diet or severe malabsorption apart from causing undernourishment and debility depresses the activity of pituitary gland producing hormonal disturbance, or a deficient diet may deprive the glands of raw material from which hormones are manufatured.

7. Finally, the constitutional causes of leucorrhoea include debilitated conditions due to anaemia, tuberculosis, etc.

In an easier and more understandable way, the causes of leucorrhoea have been described as under :-

A. **General Causes**

1. Malnutrition.
2. Sedentary habits.
3. Anaemia.
4. Chronic illness.
5. Alcohol.
6. Excess of tea and coffee.
7. Occupation : women serving the whole day long.
8. Constipation.
9. Diabetes, and
10. Intestinal worms in children.

B **Local Causes**

1. Gonorrhoea.
2. Monilia.

3. Cervical erosion.
4. Prolapse of uterus.
5. Displacements of uterus — retroversion.
6. Cancer of all types.
7. Leukoplakic vulvitis.
8. Chronic salpingits.

Causes of Leucorrhoea in Different Age Group

A. Before puberty :

1. Unhygienic conditions.
2. Gonorrhoea.
3. Worms : oxyuris verm cularis or thread worms.

B. Unmarried girls after puberty

1. Bad hygienic conditions during menses or otherwis
2. Sedentary habits.
3. Constipation.
4. Anaemia.
2. Any long continued chronic disease.
6. Congenital erosion of cervix.

C. In the married women :

1 Bad hygienic conditions.
2. Gonorrhoea.
3. Trichomonas vaginalis.
4. Monilia or fungus infection.
5. Displaced uterus--retroversion.
6. Chronic cervicitis or erosion.
7. Cancer of all types.
8. Long continued use of pessaries.
9. Repeated and excessive intercourse.
10. Birth control measures.
11. Chron health.

D. After monopause

1. Cancer of cervix.
2. Cancer of vulva.
3. Cancer of uterus.
4. Leukoplakic vulvitis.
5. Chronic cervicitis.
6. Prolapse and decubitic ulcer.
7. Gonorrhoea.
8. Trichomonas vaginalis.
9. Monilia.
10. Chronic ill-health.

Investigations :

1. History

Duration of the complaint. Childhood --Congenital erosion
After marriage -- Infection.

Gonorrhoea.

Monilia.

Trichomonas.

Excessive intercourse

About the discharge : character, modality etc.

5.**External examination** ;-- Examination of vulva : bartholin's glands, urethra, etc.

3. **Internal evaminations** :-- Examination of vagina and uterus for any inflammation, etc.

4. **Special examinations :--**

(i) Smears from urethra, vagina and cervix.

(ii) Blood examination.

(iii) Blood pressure evamination.

(iv) Urine examination.

(v) Biopsy : for evidence of malignancy.

(vi) For trichomonas, hanging drop method is done.

In order to investigate a case of leucorrhoea, the first important thing is to assess its severity, whether it is really an abnormal condition or not because, many a time a physician is consulted by an apparently worried but ignorant woman about the normal secretion. This point can be made clear by asking a few direct questions, e. g , whether clothes are soiled or not, whether it necessitates wearing of pads, etc. The physician should not take the statement of the patient as it is.

The history is important. If the discharge has appeared after marriage, gonorrhoea may be suspected. Often it dates back to the brith of a child or abortion : the cause in such cases is usually cervical erosion.

Next, enquiries are made about the nature of the discharge. Often it is possible to make a correct diagnosis by the character of the discharge. Indeed, some of the authors have classified the cause of leucorrhoea with reference to its nature. For example :--

1. Excessive discharge which is mucoid is character indicates congenital erosion, phrsiological conditions, like pregnancy and menstruation, psychosomatic conditions, like fears, anxiety etc., sexual difficulties and so on. But, it must be remembered that as acidity of the vaginal secretion is lessened by the excessive cervical secretion an infection may rapidly become established.
2. Mucopurulent discharge is invariably always due to chronic cervicitis.
3. A purulent discharge indicates in fection, the important of which are Trichomonas, Monilia and Gonarrhoea. At post-menopausal periods, it indicates senile veginitiessenile endometritis.
4. A thin discharge is an early symptom of cancer of the body of uterus which becomes offensive when infection occurs. It may also be due to hydrorrhoea—gravidarum (physiological in pregnancy).
5. Bloody leucorrhoea may indicate malignancy, cervical erosion, senile vaginities or senile endometrities.
6. Faecal discharge indicates recto-vaginal fistula; simillarly, urinary discharge indicates vescio-vaginal fistula.
7. Leucorrhoea that is irritating and causes itching is due to Trichomonas or Monilial infection.

8. The discharge which is partly watery but contains white solid masses is characteristic of monilial infection, etc., etc.

So we see how diagonosis can be made out fairly correctly by carefully observing the above mentioned points.

And then, the importance of pathological examinations of vaginal smear as an important diagnostic procedure cannot be over-stressed, as we very well, know, much information can be obtained from this about the ovarian activity, malignant conditions of the cervix and other infectians, etc.

And finally, pelvic examination, too, is very important; it is done to investigate pathological lesions. In fact, gynaecological investigation would be incomplete if pelvic examination is left.

Treatment

Almost the first impulse of many homoeopaths is to turn to their materia medica and repertory as soon as they see a case and rush to prescribe a seemingly indicated remedy only to find subsequently that they have failed miserably. The casr does not seem to respond favourably despite careful second or third prescription It happens so because there are certain factors which are responsible and which are often ignored and overlooked while treating a leucorrhoeal case. It may be due to force of habit or due to overconfidence in oneself. These factors greatly contribute to failure in homoeapathic prescribing. They can be enumerated as under .—

1. Correct diagnosis :—The first factor is to have correct diagnosis in the absence of which we cannot know what is normal or abnormal, physiological or pathological. The vaginal discharge is certainly a physiological pehnomenon of pregnancy and premenstrual congestion. In such cases, the patient does not need medication but reassurance and correct appraisal explanation of the phenomenon.

2 Mechanical factor :—One often comes across case who would not respond to the treatment until one discovers by chance that the patient has been using chemical contraceptives, intrauterine devices or pessaries too often which was a cons tant source of irritation. Unlecs their use is discontinued the physician cannot be successful in treating a case of leucorrhoea.

But sometimes, leucorrhoea is due to displacement of the uterus (as a result of congestion from twisting of the uterine blood vessels). wearing of the pessary or ring becomes essential in order to correct the malposition, alongwith the suitable medicines, diet and proper exercise. Certain factors can be held responsible to cause displacement and which should also be given proper attention e g.

(i) faulty postures,

(ii) Prolonged standing,

(iii) increased intra-abdominal pressure from lifting heavy things,

(iv) increased intra-peritoneal volume resulting from obesity and constipation.

As a matter of fact, laxity of the supporting structures is the chief cause of displacements, which develops with the advancing age and repeated pregnancies.

3 **Surgical factor** :—There are certain conditions which require the help of a surgeon, apart from mediciens, e.g., removal of pelvic adhesions or correction of some spinal abnormality, etc. etc.

4. **Dietecic errors** :—Dietetic corrections should be an important factor in the successful treatment of leucorrhoea; food toxaemias and nutritional deficiencies account for a number of diseases in the modren pattern of life, as result of constipation or chronic intestinal stasis causing leucorrhoea due to pressure of intestines upon the uterine blood vesels and thereby causing congestion of the uterus.

5. **Psychogenic factors** :—Emotional upsets often prove a constant source of mental irritations which, in turn, play an important role in causing leucorrhoea.

These are some of the important factors which often put obstacles in the way of succesful treatment of leucorrhoea. These should be removed as far as posseable. In fact, every individual case should be dealt with according to its own peculiarities.

Thus we can proceed with the treatment of leucorrhoea in the following way :—

General Treatment

(i) Rest and exercise.
(ii) Diet : non-stimulating, but nourishing.
(iii) Regularity of bowel movements and habits.
(iv) Personal hygiene is important.

Local Treatment

If the discharge is acrid and too, copious douche of normal saline water is beneficial. Otherwise, nothing is advised to apply. In some cases, Hydrastis lotion is recommended.

Medicinal Treatment

The following remedies may be given according to the symptoms, constitution and pathology as well :—

Alumina sepia, Puls., Syphilium, Borax, Kreosote, Calc. Carb., Calc. Phos, Cauloph., Cimicif Bovista, Cina, Teucrium, Dictamnus, Platina, Caust., Lil. Tig., Cocculus, Tabacum. etc.

THERAPEUTIC HINTS

Alumina :—Leucorrhoea, transparent or of yellow mucus and is profuse, acrid and excoriating, running down to the heels, with scanty, delayed and pale menses. Patient is exhausted and pale after the menses, with constipation, anaemia, craving for indigestible things like chalk, charcoal cloves and potatoes. Worse, at new and full moon. Full of fear, anxiety and confusion of mind; always in hurry ; has suicidal ideas.

Pulsatilla :—Milky leucorrhoea, which, later on, becomes watery, acrid and burning from being retained in the vagina. It is mucous, thick, creamy, white leucorrhoea, sometimes replacing menses, with chilliness, disposition to lie and lowness of spirits.

Sepia :—Leucorrhoea of yellowish green colour, somewhat offensive and often excoriating, due to pelvic congestion of a passive type. It is milky; worse before menses with bearing down; there are pains in the abdomen pruritus. Patient has a sallow, pimply face, and it is most suitable to those of dark complexion who are feeble and debilitated and who have a sensation of emptiness at pit of stomach.

Kreosote :– Leucorrhoea profuse, watery, yellow, acrid, of the odour of green corn, worse before menses and between menses Corrosive itching within the vulva with burning and swelling of Labia and things; it causes soreness and smarting and red spots and itching on the vulva, always with great debility. It is so acrid that, it causes the pudenda and thighs to swell and itch.

Borox :—Leucorrhoea like white of egg, with sensation as though hot fluid was flowing, flows down the legs and acrid in nature; midway between menses. Accompanied by other symptoms of this remedy the dread of downward motion, and mental symptoms, like anxiety, fidgetiness, sensitiveness and excessive nervouness.

Calcarea Carb :—With morning hunger, acidity of the stomach and cold and damp feet. Especially suitable to scrofulous patient with enlarged cervical glands. The leucorrhoea is profuse, milky, persitent or yellow and accomdanied by itching and burning. In infants and young girls recurring before puberty; before menses or in recurring attacks between the menses.

Arsenic :—Leucorrhoea from exhausting diseases cancer, etc. Best suited to week patients, old women, especially chronic from with much weakness; the discharge is acrid, corrosive and yellow.

Hydrastis :—Leucorrhoea acrid and corroding, shreddy and tenacious; worse, after menses; from erosion and excoriation of the cervix. Pruritus vulva with profuse leucorrhoea. Sexual excitement. Menorrhagia.

Bovista :—Leucorrhoea acried, thick, tough and greenish, after menses. Too early and profuse menses, worse at night. Cannot bear tight clothing around the waist. Diarrhoea before and during menses.

Kali Bich :—Yellow, ropy, stringy leucorrhoea. Especially suitable to fat and light-haired patients.

Lilium Tig :—Profuse excoriating, watery, yellowish or yellowish brown leucorrhoea, accompanied by a depression of spirits and bearing down in pelvic region.

Helonisas :—Profuse, yellow, thick leucorrhoea with great irritation and itching. Anemia with much prostration and general debility, worse from slight colds and exertion.

Nitric acid :—Corrosive leucorrhoea, which is greenish, offensive, and obstináte, with figwarts and condylomata.

Graphites :—With pain in lower abdomen and weakness in small of back. It is profuse, very thin, white mucus and comes out in gushis; the menses are delayed, scanty and pale. More profuse in morning when rising.

Balladonna ;—Leucorrhaea thin, odourless, bland due to pelvic idflammation and congestion; the cervix is sensitive and there are bearing down pains also.

Carbo Veg. :—Better, when the flow is on; and as soon as it disappears, other complaints appear. With other symptoms of the remedy.

Mercl. Sol. :—Acrid excoriating leucorrhoea. Smarting and burning, swelling of external genital organs. Purulent greenish yellow leucorrhoea, worse at night. Yellow and thick leucorrhoea with a history of syphilis. Itching of genitals, worse from contact of urine which must be washed with cold water immediately.

Ammon. Carb. :—Leucorrhoea burning, acrid, watery; with itching, swelling and burning of the vulva. Aversion to the other sex.

Dictamnus :—Leucorrhoea of tenacious mucus, attended with painful erosion of the external genital organs and itching of the anus.

Secale Cor. :—Brownish and offensive leucrrhoea, with metrorrhagia. Fspecially suits to the thin, scrawny women who suffer from profuse menses and prolapse.

Sulphur :—Leucorrhoea, which makes the parts sore. It is indicated more by the general symptoms, than the local ones. Discharge of all sorts, mild or excoriating; in most chronic cases, juet as in all other chronic catarrhal affections; burning of the soles of the feet, and heat in the crown of the head; too much animal heat; feeling of faintness, with strong craving for nourishment, about eleven o'clock every forenoon; vulva sore, burning and smarting.

Natrum Mur. (*Tissue remedy*) :—Leucorrhoea, a waterly scalding, irritating discharge, smarting after or between the periods. Greenish after walking, in the morning, with headache, colic, itching of vulva, and bearning down pressure. After topical application of silver nitrate.

Calcarea Phos. (*Tissue remedy*) :—Leucorrhoea, as a constitutional tonic and intercurrent with the chief remedy; a discharge of albuminous mucus. Leucorrhoea, worse after menses, looks like white of egg, with feeling of weakness in sexual organs, worse after stool and urination. Parts pulsate with voluptuous feelings. Patient takes cold readily.

Silicea (*Tissue remedy*) :—Leucorrhoea instead of menses, preceded by colicy pains, also during micturition and following obstinate constipation. Deficiency of animal heat. Especially for oversensitive, weakly women, whose constitutions are imperfectly nourished owing to deficient or imperfect assimilation.

Ammon. Mur :—Leucorrhoea with distension of the abdomen without accumulation of wind; discharge like the white of an egg, after previous pinching around the naval; brown, slimy, painless leucorrhoea, after every discharge of urine; stools hard, crumbling.

Caulophylium :—Profuse secretion of mucus in the vagina; yellowith spot on the forehead, commonly called "mooth". bearing down wita tardy or absent menses; drawing pains in the lower extremities.

Causticum :—Weakening leucorrhoea, with too scanty or too profuse menses; discharge, particularly at night; yellow face; dis inclination to coitus.

Lachesis :—Leucorrhoea before the menses, copious, smarting, slimy, stiffening and staining the linen greenish; the menses appear at the regular time, but are too short and too feeble; the abdomen is hot and tender to touch; feels bad after sleeping.

Lycopodium :—Profuse, greenish, thick discharge, not constantly, but in spells, which are always preceded by a sharp cutting pain in the hypogastrium; pale, face with frequent flushes of circumscribed redness of the cheeks; discharge of gas from the vagina; the least quantity of food fills her up to the throat; jerking of the lower extremities.

Natrum Mur. :—Leucorrhoeal discharge after contractive colic, pressing downwards, early in the morning, at night, when walking; itching and soreness of the genitals; cutting pain in the urethra after micturition; yellowness of the face; and especially after local application of nitrate of silver.

Platina :—Leucorrhoea, during daytime; genitals excessively sensitive; can't bear to be touched; will go into spasms from an examination: will almost faint during intercourse; or excessive sexual desire; haughty disposition, or low-spirited.

INFECTIONS

The female genitalia is a continuous passage extending from the vulva to the ovaries, rather the peritoneum itself, because the fimbriae, except the ovarian fimbriae, are continuation of the peritoneum. So, the infection taking place, anywhere can spread to the whole or a part of the passage. But this is not so; the infection does not take place ordinarily, because there are certain natural barriers to infection.

Vulva

The glands, wherever they are, most conducive to infection. From them, if not checked' it spreads to the lymphatics and then to the blood-stream

There are bartholin's glands which can be infected.

So, the vulva is very easily prone to infection.

Vagina.

The inner lining (stratified epithelium) of vagina can be infected; Otdinarily, infection does not take place because vaginal secretions are acidic in reaction which kill the infection unless there is a break in the vaginal walls or a change in pathology in the vaginal secretions : e. g., the secretion may be less or it may be alkaline in reaction.

So, the acidic reaction of the vaginal secretions is the natural barrier to infection in the vagina.

It is placed at a distance from the exterior and it is supplied with abundant blood supply. On account of its situation, ordinarily it is not infected from the infection in the vagina or the exterior if there is any (as it is a highly vascular organ, the infection can take place through the blood stream.) But, once the infection reaches. it is difficult to deal with it.

Uterus

It is also far away from the exterior, so, it is not easily infected unless lacerated. All the uterine infections take place at the time of and after labour.

Fallopian Tubes and Ovaries.

There are not easily infected because of their situation far away from the exterior. They get infection from the glandular structures only, when it enters the blood stream throug hthe lymphatics.

All the glandular structures are easily infected. Non-glandular structures arenot easily infected, because of the acidic vaginal secretions.

Modes of infection :

1. By spread up the lumen.
2. By lymphatic spread.
3. By blood stream.
4. By direct spread from adjacent viscera.

1, By Spread up the Lumen. -- Lumen is the tube, i e., the genital tract. It means that the infection is coming from outside ; e.g., from bartholin's glands.

Secondly PH value of and the vaginal secretion itself might be lacking. PH value of vaginal secretion is 4.5.

Every fluid is acidic or alkaline or neutral in reaction. Acidity and alkalinity of the solution depend upon the concentration of hydrogenions. PH value of water is 7, i.e.. neutrali below 7 indicates different grades of increasing acidity with O as complete acid and above 7 indicates different grades of increasing alkalinity with 14 as complete alkali

Vaginal secretion contains lactic acid, glycogen and oestrin. The female child and an old woman are more liable to infection because they have less secretion and have not sufficient amount of oestrin in vagina and also the secretion is more alkaline than acidic. So, under lack of secretions, the lady will have :

(i) Disturbed protective mechanism, and

(ii) General deibility.

Hence, she must avoid :

(i) Wearing of pessaries.

(ii) Injurious douches.

(iii) Excessive sexual intercourse : and

(iv) Instrumental attempts at abortion.

2. By Symphatic Spread :-- Wherever the glands are, they are liable to get infected and the infection travels further to the lymphatics, if not checked or treated.

3. By Blood Stream :-- The common infection reaching through the blood stream to the uterus and the fallapian tubes is the tubercular infection. The spread is, however, by th secondary infection and is very rare also.

4. By Direct Spread from Adjacent Viscera :—For example, if the appendix is infected, it can infect the genital tract, the fallopian tube in particular, by the constant touch.

Caustaive Grganism to Infection

1. Most common orgainsm is Gonococcus.
2. Less important are the pyogenic bacteria, like streptococci and staphylococci.
3. Still less important of the infections are the protozoal, fungus and tubercular infection.

Gonorrhofal infection of the Genital Tract

Gonorrhoeal infection is had in any of the following ways :--

1. Through sexual intercourse with an infected person.
2. Through contaminated hands and clothes.

The gonococci penetrate the surface between the spithelial cells and involve the superficial layer of the submucous connective tissue of the urethra producing an inflammation. Cervix, too, is mostly involved alongwith the vaginal fornices. Inflammation of batholin's glands is also present. If not checked, the infection may spread further and cause metritis, endometritis, salpingitis, oophoritis, pelvic cellulitis, pelvic peritonitis and sometimes proctitis also.

Course of Gonorrhoeai Infection

It is probable that the point of inoculation is generally some abrasion or split in the mucosa in the region of the hymen and the vaginal orifice. The inflammation spreads rapidly within the vagina and over the vulva, and it nearly always extends into the urethra. Clinically the condition is one of urethritis, vulvitis and vaginitis. In favourable cases, which constitute the majority, of course, the inflammatory process progresses no further inwards than the entrance to the cervix. In unfavourable cases, it travels up through the uterus to the fallopian tubes and to the peritoneal cavity, setting up salpingitis, pyosalpinx, and peritonitis. It is a remarkable fact that although a gonorrhoeal endometritis has been assumed as a stage in the inward progress of the disease, this condition has not been demonstrated; and some authorities hold the view that though the cervical mucosa may be actually infected, the body of the uterus acts merely as a channel by which the infection is conveyed to the fallopian tubes, and is not itself attacked.

The gonorrhoeal invasion may, therefore, be regarded clinically as consisting of two well-defined stages, the first which is more frequent and less serious being confined to the lower genital tract, and the second which is fraught with the gravest consequences being the stage in which the upper genital tract is invaded.

Gonorrhoea may invade the blood stream and produce gonorrhoeal septicaemia and thereby the metastatic effects, such as arthritis and rheumatism endocarditis, pericarditis and sometimes pelurisy.

Symptoms

Gonococcal infection produces the following symptoms :-

1. The symptoms are often so mild that the woman may not feel them at all.
2. Urinary symptoms are :--
   (i) frequency of urination. more at night.
   (ii) painful and burning sensation while passing urine.
3. Discharge of muco-purulent or purulent secretion from urethra, vagina and cervix.

4. Inflammation of vulva, vagina and cervix.
5. General sympotms, like
   (i) fever
   (ii) headache
   (iii) restlessness
   (iv) loss of appetite, and
   (v) loss of sleep.
6. Increased vaginal discharge which may be due to coexisting vaginal parasite -- trichomonas voginalis.
7. Sometimes, there may be acute erosion of the cervix.
8. Besides all this, gonorrhoea may produce above said complications.

— —

CHAPTER XVIII

DISEASES OF THE VULVA

Vulvitis

VULVITIS means the infection of vulva causing inflammation. It may be acute or chronic.

Aetiology

The causes of actute vulvitis may be enumerated as under :–

1. Gonococci.
2. Streptococci.
3. Protozoa.
4. Fungus.

1. Gonorrhoeal infection :—Wherever the inflammation is, four cardinal sings are present :—

(i) Heat, i.e., fever,

(ii) Redness,

(iii) Swelling, and

(iv) Pain.

Other symptoms are :—

(v) Urethritis because infection invades the urethra also alongwith the vulva.

(vi) Pain during micturition, if there is an injury.

(vii) If the infection goes further, it causes bubo, i.e., the inguinal glands are inflamed.

(iiiv) And, after that, there is the purulent yellowish greenish discharge.

Diagnosis

Four cardinal symptoms of inflammation are present. Urethra is as a cord like structure lying over the vaginal wall ; we

squeeze out some discharge from it and send it to the pathologist for examination to find out the specific organism.

Treatment

Modern allopathic treatment is, however, penicillin or other antibiotics. Gonorrhoea is actually an infection of the urethra.

Homoeopathic Remedies

Puls., Ars., Copaiva, Hydras., Merc. Sol., Thuja, Medorrhinum, Apis, Canth., Can. Sat., Dulc., China.

2. **Streptococcal infection** :—It is also known as membranous vulvitis. Streptococus is very very violent and thus causes necrosis. Then it will look like a yellowish greenish discharge as the pus is present : Four sings of inflammation with areas of necrosis having sloughs.

Vulvitis may also be due to diphtheria becillus called Klebb's Leoffler's becillus. The difference, clinically, is that the diphtheria cases are more toxic, membrane is of greenish colour and is adherent, if we try to remove the septic patches, they are not easily removed and will cause pain and bleeding.

Treatment

Local :—Paint the vulva with 1% gentian violet lotion to soothe the irritation.

Hemoeopathic remedies

Ars., Borax. Carbo Veg., Merc. Sol., Sul. Ac., Nit. ac., Nat, Mur., Kali Mur , Kali Bich., Kreosote, Sepia and Thuja.

3. **Protozoal infection** :—Protoral vulvitis occurs only where the protozoa are abundant. This variety is not very common and is prevalent mostly in the coastal areas.

Four signs of inflammation plus periodicity to protozoa, as is in malaria : of course, only pathological tests will show the protozoal infection.

Treatment

Treatment is the same in almost all the varieties of vulvities.

Homoeopathic remedies

As periodicity is marked in the protozoal type of valvities, we can think of all the medicines which have periodicity in their symptomatology; like, Ars., China, China ars., China Sul., Natr. Mur., Arg Met., Alumina, Ipecac, Sepia, Silicea, etc.

4. **Fungus infections** :—It is also known as aphthous vulvitis occuring as a result of fungus—commonly due to candida—albicans.

It causes typical small white blisters on the vulva--over the thighs.

It is very less common because it occurs after menopause mostly.

Treatment

Paint the vulva with 1% gentian violent solution to soothe the irritation.

If vulvitis occurs in pregnancy when there is glycosurea, it is usually due to diabetes and in pruritus. So, check the urine for sugar also, in case of fungus infection.

Control diabetes with diet and suitable medicines.

Homoeopathic remedies

Helonias, Ars., Borax, Merc. Sol., Sulph. acid, Carbo Veg., Nat. Mur., Nit. acid, Kreosote, Kali Bich., Kali Mur., Sepia, Thuja and others according to symptoms.

THERAPEUTIC HINTS

Arsenic :—Itching, burning, pain as from red, hot wires; worse least exertion; causes great weakness; feels better in warm room, warmth. With great restlessness, anxiety and fear, thirsty for small quantity of water at short intervals. Periodicity is marked. The infection may be of streptococcal, protozoal or fungus origin.

Belladonna :—Great heat, redness and burning of the part; acute inflammation with suddenness of its onset. Dryness. Pain with sensitiveness of the vulva. Patient wants to be quiet; feels worse by touch and movement, jar,

Merc. Sol. :—Eruptions with itching and burning, worse after urinating, better washing with cold water; worse at night, from warmth of bed, during perspiration. Parts are much swollen. with raw, sore feeling. Tendency to pus formation; streptococcal or fungus infection. History of syphilis or gonorrhoea is often present.

Thuja :—History of gonorrhoea is traced, with condylomata and warty excrescences on the vulva and perineum. Burning during micturition.

Borax :—Aphthous patches on the vulva with itching. Of use in aphthous vulvitis occuring as a result of fungus infection. Dread of downward motion is prominently present.

Carbo Veg. :—Septic condition with burning sensation. Vulva sowllen; aphthous patches and distended veins on the vulva. Itching, worse in evening, when warm in bed. The discharge is offensive.

Sulphuric acid :—Streptococcal and fungus vulvitis. Hot flushes followed by perspiration. Wants everything to be done in a hurry. Vulvitis after some mechanical injury.

Nitric acid :—Blisters and ulcers on the vulva, which bleed easily; with soreness. Hair fall off. History of syphilis or abuse of mercury may be traceable. Sticking pains; pain as from splinters. Especially suitable in dark complexioned patients who are past middle life.

Natrum Mur. :—Great weakness and weariness. Oversensitive to all sorts on influences. Depressed state of mind. Consolation aggravates. Dry eruptions in the groins, with itching, burning rawness, and redness. Craving for salt is very great and it seems probable that the condition is due to the intake of salt in excess. Protozoal infection; marked periodicity.

Kali Mur. :—This is a tissue remedy, used more or less empirically for all infective processes, like penicillin in the other school of medicine. History of syphilis or gonorrhoea. Alongwith it, cystitis is also met with where the discharge is thick, white mucus.

Kali Bich: :—Vulvitis associated with pruritus, with great burning and excitement; worse in hot weather. Especially indicated in fleshy, fat, light complexioned patients subject to catarrhs or with syphilitic or scrofulous history. With ulcers, especially punched out ulcers; the discharge, if present, is tough, stringy and viscid.

Kali Carb. :—Sharp and cutting pains. Weakness is pronounced, with backache relieved by sitting and pressure. Vulvitis occuring after parturition. Genitals feel sore; with pains from back pass down through gluteal muscles.

Kreosote :—Post menopausal vulvitis; with corrosive itching and burning and swelling of labia; with violent itching between labia and thighs. Burning and soreness in the vulva. Leucorrhoea is yellow, acrid, and of the smell of green corn.

Sepia :—A very good menopausal remedy, and otherwise also. Streptococcal or fungus infection. Hot flushes at menopause with weakness and perspiration. Among the mental symptoms, lack of affection is important. With prolapse of the uterus and violent stitches upward in vagina and bearing down.

Helonias :—Sensation of weakness, dragging and weight in the sacrum and pelvis; with profund melancholia. Pruritus; the vulva is hot, red, swollen, with terrible burning and itching.

Pulsatilla :—With history of gonorrhoea. Commencement of the affection dates back to the age of puberty; or the affection at menopause. Weeps easily; of mild and yielding nature. Pain in back with tried feeling.

Apis :—Swelling, itching, burning of the vulva with stinging pains, better by washing with cold water. Sense of tightness; with bearing down, as if the menses would appear.

Cathanris :—Violent inflammation with hypersensitiveness; black swelling of the vulva with irritation. Raw, burning pain. Accompanied by dysuria, intolerable frequent urgings to pass urine.

Cannabis Sativa :—Gonorrhoeal vulvitis ; with urethra sensitive and burning while urinating, extending to bladder.

Dulcamara :—Inflammation from cold and dampnese; as a result of sudden change of weather when the days are hot and the nights cold towards the close of summer; from living or working in damp, cold besements. Follicular, herpetic vulvitis.

China :—Debility. Periodicity is most marked. With painful heaviness in the pelvic region.

Copaiva :—With itching of the vulva and anus, and swelling of urethral orifice, dysuria, and a constant desire to urinate.

Hydrastis :—With leucorrhoea, worse after menses; acrid and corroding, shreddy and tenacious; pruritus.

Medorrhinum :—Intense pruritus. Leucorrhoea, thin, acrid, excoriating and of fishy smell. Sycotic warts on the genitals. Suppressed gonorrhoeal history.

Asafoetida :—Syphilitic origin; with extreme sensitiveness and night pains.

Colcarea Carb :—Burning and itching with much sweat about the external genitals. Early and profuse menses. In fat, fair and flabby patients. Glands in the groins swollen. It is a great antipsoric remedy.

Coccus Cacti :—Inflammation of labia, with dysuria and heamaturia and, as a result of urinary calculi.

Merc. Cor :—Vulvities, with tenesmus of the rectum and the bladder as well. Gonorrhoea, second stage. Intense burning in urethra; urine hot, burning scanty, or even suppressed, bloody, greenish, and albumen mixed.

Petroleum :—Genitals sore, with sensation of moisture. Profuse and albuminous leucorrhoae.

— —

CHAPTER XIX
PRURITUS VULVA

PRURITUS-VULVA is the inflammation and itching of the vulval area.

Aetiology

1. Mainly diabetes; it is the most important cause.
2. Protozoal infection, especially Trichomonas.
3. Fungus infection.
4. Discharge from the cervix, especially gonorrhoeal.
5. Dischrage caused by neglected pessaries or vesico-vaginal fistula (the urine causes irritation).
6. Thread-worms in children.
7. Eczema around it will cause pruritis.
8. Toxaemia during pregnancy.
9. Premenstrual congestion.
10. Deficiency of ovarian hormones with atrophy of external genitals.
11. In many cases, no cause is found, where diet and unhygienic habits of living are considered to be the causing factor.

Signs and Symptoms

1. Itching and irritation, more in the night.
2. Disturbed and loss of sleep.
3. When there is a syphilitic taint, there is suicidal tendency.

Labia-minora and clitoris are usually attacked first.

Treatment

1. Find out the cause by laboratory findings and treat accordingly.

2. Hot water bottles may be applied for soothing purpo ses.

3. If no cause is found, apply some local application : Hydorcortisone ointment is very good (in allopathy). Homoeopathic lotions are good : Urtica urens, Cantharis, calend ula, Apis, etc.

4. X-ray treat ment is also recommended by the modern school.

5. Hormonal treatment, too is often beneficial. Oestrin can be given.

6. *Homoeopathic remedies*

Ambra Grisea. Canth., Fagopyrum, Radium Brom., Tarentula, Hisp., Sulphur. Ars., Sepia, Carboveg and other medicine according to the symptoms.

7. In severe cases, put the lady on milk diet for few days.

THERAPEUTIC HINTS

Ambra Grisea :—Itching during pregrancy, with soreness and swelling of the parts; nymphomania. Numb feeling of the whole body surface in the morning; perspiration of the abdomen and thighs in the daytime when moving about; falling out of the hair, and great sensitiveness of the scalp to the touch. Menses are early. Profuse, bluish leucorrhoea. Patient wants to be alone, she is afraid of the presence of other people. Music is unbearable for her. It is especially useful for those who are thin, scrawny and hysterical and for those also who are weakened by age or overwork. An excellent old age remedy.

Arsenic :—Itching with great burning and probably swelling also, better by heat and warmth; and attended by much restlessness, anxiety and werkness. It is good for chronic cases. Itching is worse by cold and scrathing.

Cantharis :—Violent itching, with inflammation and burning, and sexual mania; nymphomania. Black swelling of vulva with irritation. Often attended by urethrities, with painful micturition.

Carbo Veg :—Vulva is swollen. Leucorrhoea, thick, greenish milky, excoriating, worse before menses. The menses are premature and too profuse; pale blood. There is burning in hands and soles during menses. Itching is worse in evening, when warm in bed.

Sepia :—Itching from leucorrhoea, which is yellow, greenish. Irregular menses; late and scanty or early and profuse; with sharp cutting pains. Prolapse of the uterus and vagina, from laxity of the organs. Bearing down sensation as if everything would come out through the vulva ; must cross the legs to prevent it. Dyspareunia. Plus other symptoms of the remedy.

Sulphur :—Severe itching with burning ; scratching aggravates ; the parts get red, sore and burning. The menses are late, scanty, short and difficult ; are thick, black and acrid, making the parts sore. Leucorrhoea, burning, and excoriating. When an indicated remedy fails to give its desired effect or as a terminating remedy to complete the cure

Radium Brom. :—Itching worse in bed or in warmth ; with aching pains in abdomen over the pubes during the flow of menses. The menses are delayed and irregular, with backache. Itching attended by severe aching pains all over, with restlessness, better by moving about. Right breast is sore, relieved by rubbing it hard.

Tarentula Hispania :—Vulva is dry and hot, with much itching, nymphomania. The complaints attended by extreme restlessness; so much so that she feels like keeping in constant motion, even though walking aggravates.

Fagopyrum :—Pruritus, with yellow leucorrhoea, worse rest, scratching and touch ; and better by bathing in cold water. Pruritus senilis.

Helonias :—The parts are hot, red and swollen ; they burn and itch terribly Dragging and pain in sacral region, with prolapse, especially after miscarriage ; she is very conscious of her uterus. Menses, here, are too frequent and profuse. Albuminuria.

Hydrastis :-Itching with profuse leucorrhoea, which is acride and corroding, shreddy and tenacious and worse after menses. Erosion and excoriation of the cervix. Attended by sexual excitement, dull, heavy dragging pain and stiffness, especially across lumbar region, compelling her to use the arms in rising from the seat.

Croton Tig :—Intense itching, but scratching is very painful. Pustular eruption on the external genitalia with great itching, followed by painful burning.

Conium :—Itching around the pudenda ; rash before menses. The menses are delayed and scanty, and the parts are sensitive. With weakness of the body and mind.

Caladium :—Itching of the vulva and vagnia during pregnancy ; with voluptuousness, sometimes causing the habit or onanism. Dread from motion is marked.

Calcarea Carb :—Itching and burning of the parts before and after menses ; in little girls. Much sweating about the external genitalia. Increased sexual desire ; easy conception ; or sterility with copious menses. The typical constitution of Calcarea is present; fair, fat and flabby with much perspiration.

Graphites :—Fat, chilly and costive patient, with delayed menstrual history, and a tendency to skin affections and constipation ; and who are stout, of fair complexion and take cold easily. Itching of the vulva, before menses ; they are late, pale and scanty, with tearing pain in the epigastrium ; leucorrhoea is pale, thin, white, and excoriating.

Kreosote :—Corrosive itching within the vulva, with burning and swelling of labia ; violent itching between the labia and thighs. Eruption appears after menses. Burning and soreness in external and internal parts. Leucorrhoea yellow acrid ; of the odour of green corn ; worse between periods.

Mercurius :—Itching and burning, worse after urination, better by washing the parts with cold water. Leucorrhoea, excoriating, greenish and bloody ; with sensation of rawness in the parts and stinging pain in the ovaries. Plus, the general characteristics of mercury.

Rhus Tox :—Swelling with intense itching of the vulva ; worse, cold, wet rainy weather and after rains, at night, during rest.

Medorrhinum :—Intense itching Leucorrhoea thin, acrid, excoriating and of fishy odour. History of sycosis is generally present. In sterile women. —

CHAPTER XX

BARTHOLINITIS

BARTHOLINITIS means an inflammation of the bartholin's glands.

They are two in number situated on either side of the vaginal orifice on the vaginal surface by small ducts just below and anterior to the hymen.

Aetiology

1. Mostly gonorrhoeal infection.
2. Puerperal infection.
3. Obstruction of the duct due to cyst or calculus formation.

A piece of stone from the urethra may get imbedded. The cysts appear on the posterior burrow deep into the posterior labial wall.

There may be no symptoms or discomfort, but when infected, they may cause discomfort.

Differential Diagnosis

This condition should be differentially diagnosed from :—

1. Inguinal hernia, and
2. Haematoma.
3. Cyst.
4. Abscess., and
5. Malignancy of the inguinal glands.

Treatment

If the pus has formed, it has to be aspirated and then calendula lotion should be applied.

2. When the cause is gonorrhoea, the treatment should be on the gonorrhoeal lines.

3. If calculus is imbedded in the gland or the duct, it has to be taken out by excision.

4. Excision of the gland and duct is to be resorted to when malignancy is suspected or has taken place.

5. *Homoeopathic remedies*

Ars., Bell., Hepar Sulph , Silicea. Merc. Sol., Net. acid, Kreosote, Sepia, Thuja and Medorrhinum.

THERAPEUTIC HINTS

Arsenic :—Inflammation with burning, pain, better by heat and warmth; restlessness, anxiety and fear and great prostration. Leucorrhoea is acrid, burning, offensive and thin. Pain is felt as from red hot wires, worse least exertion ; causes great weakness ; and she is better in a warm room.

Apis Mel. :—Soreness and burning stinging pains, with oophoritis, oedema of labia, better by cold water. Dysmenorrhoea, with severe ovarian pains, and a sense of tighteness.

Belladonna :—Acute inflammation, with sudden onset, dryness and heat of the vagina, cutting, throbbing pains; worse, least motion, jar and touch.

Hepar Sulph. :—Inflammation, with extreme tenderness and pain threatening pus-formation, with itching of pudenda, worse cold, touch and motion.

Silicea :—Inflammation with pus-formation. Milky, cyst-formation. Milky, acrid leucorrhoea, during urination ; itching of vulva and vagina. Patient is very chilly ; she is worse by cold in any form.

Mercurius :—Inflammation with stinging pain in ovaries, itching, and buning, worse at night, in bed ; better by cold washing. Syphilitic history may be traced. Patient perspires greatly. The inflammation may threaten pus also.

Nitric Acid :—External parts sore, with ulcers, which bleed easily ; splinter-like pains. Worse, evening and night ; better while riding in a carriage.

Kreosote :—Very severe and old neuralgic pains, worse by rest ; with excoriating, burning and offensive discharge and violent itching.

Sepia :—Prolapse condition of the uterus and vagina. Violent stitches upward in vagina. Bearing down sensation is very marked. Indifferent to the loved ones, household work and her occupation even. Leftsided gland is generally involved

Thuja :—History of gonorrhoea may be traced. Warty growth. Vagina is very painful. Tearing pain in the glands. very sensitive to touch.

Medorrhinum :—Condition occuring after suppressed gonorrhoea. For women who suffer from chronic pelvic disorders. The pains are intolerable and tensive ; the nerves quiver and give tingling sensation. Time passes slowly for her ; has fear of dark and of someone behind her.

CHAPTER XXI

DISEASES OF THE VAGINA

ACUTE VAGINITIS

ACUTE VAGINITIS means an acute inflammation of the vaginal mucosa.

Aetiology

It may occur due to any of the following causes :—

1. Injury to vagina during labour.

2. Injury by too hot douches or introduction of foreign bodies or instruments.

3. Gonococci, mainly responsible for vaginitis.

Signs and Symptoms

1. **Congestion** :—As more of blood reaches the vaginal epithelium to fight out the infecting agent, congestion occurs.

2. **Heat** :—The vaginal walls become hotter alongwith the raised body temperature on account of bacterial activity.

3. **Swelling** :—It takes place after the incoming of more blood in the mucous membrane of vagina.

4. **Pain** :—Pain is due to irritation of the sensory nerves.

5. **Dyspareunia** :—It means painful intercourse occuring due to the acute inflammation.

6. **Discharge** :—The discharge is of greenish mucopurulent matter.

7. **Vaginal wall** :—The wall of vagina will show red indurated nodules.

Treatment

General :

1. Find out the cause and treat accordingly. (Send the pus matter or the disrharge for the examination of bacterial infection).

2. Discontinue the use of pessaries if she is using any, because the pessary causes constant irritation.

Local :

Usually, in cases of vaginal infections, P.H. is altered. P.H. is generally high or raised ; so, give lactic acid douche with 2% solution to bring the P.H. to normal, thereby killing the bacteria.

In pyogenic infections, P.H. is 6–7. In protozoal and gonorrhoeal infections, P.H. is between 5 and 6.

Medicinal :

Aco., Apis, Bell., Ganth., Croton Tig., Helonias Hydrastis, Kreosote, Merc. C; Sepia, Puls.

THERAPEUTIC HINTS

Aconite :—Acute inflammation with sudden and violent onset, and with great anxiety and fear of death. The attack is so severe that she predicts the time of her death. History of exposure to dry cold winds in winter or to heat of very hot weather in plethoric women. Vagina is dry, hot and sensitive.

Apis Mellifica :—Burning and stinging pains with oedema of the labia, better by cold water. Dysmenorrhoea, with sense of tightness and bearing down, as if the menses would appear. Pain is worse by heat, slightest touch, in the afternoon and after sleep. The patient is very jealous, tearful, fidgety and hard to please.

Belladonna :—Sudden and acute inflammation, with heat, redness, throbbing and burning in vagina. Vagina is dry and hot; dragging around the loins and pain in secrum. Sensitive forcing downwords as if all to the organs would protrude. Alongwith it, there is rush of blood to the face and head, so that she has blood shot eyes with congested face and throbbing headache.

Cantharis :—Raw burning pains and intolerable, constant urging to pass urine ; the act of urination is painful. Urine scalds her, and is passed drop by drop ; there is cutting pain before, during and after the urine. Nymphomania ; the menses are early and profuse ; black swelling of the vulva with irritation.

Croton Tig. :—Inflammation and irritation; with the formation of vesicles and mucous discharge from the vagina.

Helonias :—Profound melancholia prevales all through; and she feels better when she keeps herself busy in doing something. The vagina is hot and red; burns and itch terribly. There is a sensation of weakness, dragging and weight in the sacral region and in the pelvis, with great languor and prostration. Vaginitis with pruritus vulva.

Hydrastis :—Vaginitis from erosion and excoriation of the cervix ; leucorrhoea, acrid and corroding, shreddy and tenacious. There is dull, heavy, dragging pain and stiffness, especially, across the lumber region, so that she must use her arms in raising herself from the seat. Pruritus and sexual excitement accompany.

Kreosote :—With great burning and swelling of the labia, and corrosive itching within the vulva. There is burning and soreness in the external and internal genital organs. Leucorrhoea, yellow, acrid and of the smell of green corn. There is dragging backache, extending to the genitals and down the thighs, with great debility.

Merc. Cor. :—Tenesmus is present all through ; of the rectum, bladder and genitals. Gonorrhoea, in its second stage; or a history of syphilis or gonorrhoea is traced. Aggravation at night and during perspiration, which is usually very profuse, heat, especially heat of the bed. There is itching and burning in the vagina, worse after urination, so that, she must wash the parts with cold water.

Sepia :—Violent stitches upward in the vagina, from the uterus to the umbilicus. Vagina is very painful, especially during intercourse. Bearing down sensation is very marked, so she feels like crossing her legs or to press against the vulva to prevent the protrusion while sitting. There is weakness in the small of back ; and the pains extend into the back. The patient is very sad, tearful, irritable and indifferent to her own people.

——

CHAPTER XXII
TRICHOMONAS VAGINITIS

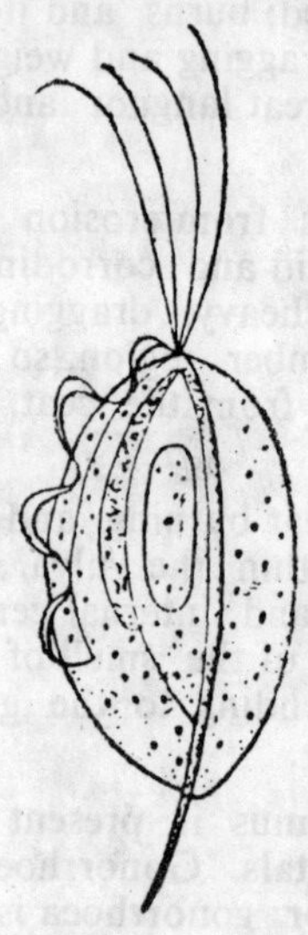

The cause here is the protozoal infection. (tricho means protozoa). The organism responsible is Trichomonas-vaginalis.

Signs and Symptoms

1. Offensive irritating discharge.
2. Dysareunia.
3. Pruritus.
4. Vulva is also involved, so that it is red and inflamed.
5. Extension of dermatitis to the thighs.

Diagnosis

First is the clinical examination and then order for the pathological examination of the v ginal smear for the presence of protozoa.

While taking the discharge as a specimen for examination, do not use any lubricant on your finger, because the protozoa may lose their motility in the lubricant and that they are recognized by their motility.

Treatment

Some arsenic preparations (such as Desulin tablets) are being used in order to kill the protozoa, by the practitioners in modern medicine. It contains arsenic, boric and glycerine.

1. Insert two tablets each night for a week ; then one tablet, till the menses start ; and then a course of 10 days.
2. Douching with 1% lactic acid.
3. After all, the indicated homoeopathic remedies depending upon the totality of characteristic symptoms, constitution caustion :

   Calc. C., Kreosote, Merc., Puls., Sepia, Thuja and the remedies given under vaginitis.

THERAPEUTIC HINTS

Calcarea Carb :—Leucophlegmatic constitution; the patient is fat, fair flabby and perspiring and chilly. Increased sexual desire ; and easy conception. Vaginitis, with much sweat about the external genitals ; sterility with profuse menses. Pain in back, as if sprained ; can scarcely rise from the seat; pain from overlifting. Weakness in small of back.

Kreosote :—Vaginitis with great burning and swelling of the labia and corrosive itching within the vulva. There is burning and soreness in the external and internal genital organs. Lecorrhoea, yellow, acrid, and of the odour of green corn. There is dragging backache extending to the genitals and down the thighs, with great debility.

Mercurius :—History of syphilis or gonorrhoea is often traced ; or even in their active stage. Inflammation with a tendency to pus-formation, which is thin, greenish and putrid. There is itching and burning in the vagina and vulva, worse after urination ; so much so, that she must wash the parts with cold water. Aggravation, at night, heat, especially heat of the bed, during perspiration which is usually very profuse. With bruised pain in small of back, especially on sitting ; tearing pain in coccyx, better by pressing on the abdomen.

Pulsatilla :--Complaints occuring from getting feet wet. The menses are late, scanty, thick, dark, clotted, changeable and intermittent, with chilliness, nausea, downward pressure and pain. Leucorrhoea acrid, burning and of creamish colour. Pain in back with a tired feeling. Attended with dyspeptic symptoms and thirstlessness. The patient is of mild, gentle and yielding disposition ; tearful, even when talking, she seeks open air and always feels better there even though she is chilly. Changeability of symptoms is marked under this remedy.

Sepia :—Violent stitches upward in the vagina, from the uterus to the umbilicus. Vagina is very painful, especially during intercourse. Bearing down sensation is very marked, so she feels like crossing her legs, or to press against the vulva to prevent the protrusion, while sitting. There is weakness in the small of back ; and the pains extend into the back. The patient is very sad, tearful, irritable and indifferent to her own people.

Thuja :—A great remedy for diseases of the genital organs. Hydrogenoid constitution. The vagina is very sensitive. Warty growths on the vulva and perineum. Profuse leucorrhoea, thick and greenish. Severe pain in the left ovary and left inguinal region. Worse at night, from heat of bed, from cold damp air. The patient has fixed ideas ; feels as if a strange person were at her side.

CHAPTER XXIII
SENILE VAGINITIS

It is a very mild variety of vaginitis and is usually met with after menopause.

Aetiology

1. Oestrin deficiency :

   Oestrin is a secretion from the ovaris and it is important for the growth of endometrium and vaginal lining. So, when it is deficient, it causes thining down of the vaginal lining and the endometrium,

2. Other causes may be any of those mentioned under vaginitis.

Signs and Symptoms

1. Purulent vaginal discharge.
2. Intermitent bleeding.
3. On examination, vagina shows granular red appearance.
4. Desquamation (peeling off) of the vaginal epithelium. There will be ulcers and healing by the fibrous tissue. So, the contraction or narrowing of the vagina takes place. Sometimes, the walls of vagina get adhered together.
5. Adherent surfaces.

Treatment

1. To increase the vaginal epithelium, stilboestrol (containing oestrin) .5 mgm. is to be given for several days. As the secretion of oestrin by the ovaries is stopped after menopause, according to the substitution theory this function is taken by the adrenal glands ; but, that is only temporary. Then, there may be some defect in the functioning of any of the endocrinal glands.
2. Lactic acid douche with 1% solution.

3. Then, treat the patient constitutionally.

Most important drugs for post menopansal complications are Sepia and Lachesis.

Others remedies being :

Aco., Apis, Rell., Canth., Croton Tig., Helon., Hydrastis, Kreosote, Merc, Puls., Calc. Carb., Thuja, Medo., etc.

THERAPEUTIC HINTS

Aconite :—Acute inflammation with sudden and violent onset, and with great anxiety and fear of death. The attack is so severe that she predicts the time of her death. History of exposure to dry cold winds in winter or to heat of very hot weather in plethoric women. Vagina is dry, hot and sensitive.

Apis Mellifica :—Burning and sitinging pains with oedema of the labia better by cold water. Dysmenorrhoea. Sense of tightness and bearing down sensation, as if the menses would appear. Pain is worse by heat, sightest touch, in the afternoon, and after sleep. The patient is very jealous, tearful, fidgety and hard to please.

Belladonna ;—Sudden and acute inflammation, with heat, redness, throbbing and burning in vagina. Vagina is dry and hot; dragging around the loins and pain in sacrum. Sensitive forcing downwards as if all the organs would protrude. Alongwith it, there is rush of blood to the face and heat, so that she has blood shot eyes with congested face and throbbing headache.

Calcarea Carb :—Leucophlegmatic constitution; the patient is fat, fair, flabby and perspiring and chilly. Increased sexual desire; and easy conception. Vaginitis, with much sweat about the external genitals; sterility with profuse menses. Pain in back, as if sprained; can scarcely rise from the seat; pain from overlifting. Weakness in small of back.

Cantharis :—Raw burning pains and intolerable, constant urging to pass urine; the act of urination is painful. Urine scalds her, and is passed drop by drop; there is cutting pain before, during and after the urine. Nymphomania; the menses are early and profuse; black swelling of the vulva irritation.

Conium :—An excellent remedy for old age, especially for old maids, who have difficult gait, termbling, sudden loss of strength while walking, painful stiffness of the legs, hypochondriasis, urinary troubles, weakned memory and sexual debility. Mammae lax and shrunken, hard and painful to touch; stitches in nipples; the patient wants to press the breast hard with hands Itching around pudenda. As a result of the repressed sexual desire or from excessive indulgence. With dull aching pain in the lumbar and sacral regions.

Croton Tig. :—Inflammation and irritation; with the formation vesicles and mucous discharge from the vagina.

Helonias :—Profound melancholia prevails all through; and she feels better when she keeps her busy in doing something. The vagina is hot and red; burns and itch terribly. There is a sensation of weakness, dragging and weight in the sacral region and in the pelvis with great lanquor and prostration, Vaginities with pruritus vulva.

Hydrastis :—Vaginities from erosion and excoriation of the cervix; leucorrhoea, acrid and corroding, shreddy and tenacious. There is dull, heavy, dragging pain and stiffness, especially, across the lumber region, so that she must use her arms in raising herself from the seat. Pruritus and sexual excitement accompany.

Kreosote :—With great burning and swelling of the labia, and corrosive itching within the vulva. There is burning and soreness in the external and internal genital organs. Leucorrhoea, yellow, acrid and of the smell of green corn. There is dragging backache, extending to the genitals and down the thighs, with great debility.

Lachesis :—Raw burning pains and intolerable urging to pass urine; the act of urination is painful. Urine scalds her and is passed drop-by-drop; there is cutting pain before, during and after the urine. Nymphomania; the menses are early and profuse; black swelling of the vulva with irritation. Flushes of heat with hypersensitivity to pressure and contact of clothes on the abdomen and waist. The patient is highly jealous, locquacious and afraid of the dark.

Lycopodium :—Carbo-nitrogenoid constitution. Affects more on the right side; or the disease travels from the right to the left side and is worse in the evening, from about 4-8 P.M. Attended with the digestive disturbances. The complaints develop gradually. The patient is thin, withered, full of gas and dry; craves everything warm; is melancholic, and afraid to be alone. The vagina is dry; coition is painful; with varicose veins of the pudenda; leucorrhoea is acrid, with burning in vagina; and bleeding from the genitals during stool; pain in the small of back accompanies.

Medorrhinum :—From suppressed gonorrhoea; for women with chronic pelvic disorders. The pains are intolerable and tensive; as if the nerves quiver and give a tingling sensation. Vaginitis with intense itching; a sensitive spot near the os. Leucorrhoea is thin, acrid, excoriating and of fishy odour. Sterile women. The breasts are cold, sore and sensitive to touch. Pain in back with burning and heat; legs heavy, and they ache the whole night, she cannot keep them still; burning of hands and feet with soreness. Worse, during day (sunrise to sunset), and heat; better by lying on the abdomen. The memory becomes weak; the patient loses the thread of conversation; the time passes very slowly for her; has fear of the dark and of some one behind her.

Mercurius :—History of syphilis or gonorrhoea is often state traced; or even in their active state. Inflammation with a tendency to pus-formation, which is thin, greenish and putrid. There is itching and burning in the vagina and vulva, worse after irrination; so much so, that she must wash the parts with cold water. Aggravation, at night, heat, especially heat of the bed, during perspiration which is usually very profuse. With bruised pain in small of back, especially on sitting; tearing pain in coccyx, better by pressing on the abdomen.

Oophorinum :—Indicated for climacteric disturbances generally, or after oophorectomy.

Pulsatilla :—Complaints occuring from getting feet wet. The menses are late, scanty, thick, dark, clotted, changeable and intermittent, with chilliness, nausea, downward pressure and pain. Leucorrhoea acrid, burning and of creamish colour. Pain in back with a tired feeling. Attended with dyspeptic symptoms and thirstlesseness. The patient is of mild, gentle and yielding disposition; tearful, even when talking; she seeks open air and always feels better there even though she is chilly. Changeability of symptoms is marked under this remedy.

Sepia :—Violent stitches upward in the vagina, from the uterus to the umbilicus. Vagina is very painful, especially during intercourse. Bearing down sensation is very marked, so she feels like crossing her legs or to press against the vulva to prevent the protrusion While sitting these is weakness in the small of back; and the pains extend into the back. The patient is very sad, tearful, irritable and indifferent to her own people.

Thuja :—A great remedy for diseases of the genital organs. Hydrogenoid constitution. The vagina is very sensitive. Warty growths on the vulva and perineum. Profuse leucorrhoea, thick and greenish. Severe pain in the left ovary and left inguinal region. Worse at night, from head of bed, from cold damp air. The patient has fixed ideas; feels as if a strange person were at her side.

CHAPTER XXIV

MICOTIC VAGINITIS

It is also known as *Vaginal Thrush.*

Aetiology

The cause is the fungus infection, especially Candida Albicans.

Signs and Symptoms

1. Thick cheesy discharge.
2. Vulva and vagina are sore and tender.

This condition is usually found in old ladies, because the vaginal secretion is less and the P.H. is higher. The fungus grows in vaginal P H. 5 and also at places where glucose is present

3. So, glycosurea is the cause.

Treatment

1. Clean the vagina with normal saline.
2. Paint the vagina with 2% acquous solution of Gentian violt or horroeopathic solutions of Hydratis, Silicea, etc.
3. *Homoeopathic remedies* :

Aco., Bell., Ars., Rhus Tox., Borax, Ambra Gr., Helon., Kreosote, Canth., Apis, Merc., Natr. Mur., Kali Mur., Kali Bich., Hydras., Sepia, Sulph., Thuja, Medo , and Nitr. acid.

In such infections, the discharge is generally bland, thick and greenish ; so, fungus are to be given ; such as :

Ars., Natr Mur., Canth, Borax, and Nitr. acid.

THERAPEUTIC HINTS

Arsenic :—Debility, exhaustion, and restlessnes ; night aggravation of the symptoms ; with fear, fright and worry. Inflammation and swelling of the genitals, with dryness of the vagina ; burning pains, better by warmth ; unquenchable thirst, drinks often but little at a time. Pain as from red-hot wires, worse by least exertion and which causes great fatigue. Weakness in small of back, with pain and burning.

Borax :—Dread of dawnward motion is present all through. Aphthous patches, and ulcerations in the vagina ; white fungus like growth ; these ulcers bleed on being touched. Pruritus of the vulva and eczema. Menses too soon, profuse, with griping, nausea and pain in stomach extending into the small of back. In sterile women.

Cantharis :—Raw, burning pains and introlerable, constant urging to pass urine ; the act of urination is painful. Urine scalds her and is passed drop-by-drop ; there is cutting pain before, during and after the urine. Nymphomania the menses are early and profuse ; black swelling of the vulva with irritation.

Natrum Mur. :—Dryness of the vagina ; the menses are irregular, but are usually profuse. Leucorrhoea acrid, watery. Bearing down pains, worse in the morning. Urine is increased and involuntary when walking, or coughing, etc She has to wait a long time for it to pass if others are present. Ill-effects of long lasting grief; she is depressed, but the consolation aggravates.

Nitric acid :—With blisters and ulcers and stitches through the vagina. External parts sore with ulcers; hair fall out. Leucorrhoea brown, flesh coloured, watery, or stringy and offensive. The menses are profuse and like muddy water, with pain in back, hips and thighs. The urine is very offensive and smells like horse's urine. Has history of syphilis or gonorrhoea. Amelioration of the symptoms while riding in a carriage.

— —

CHAPTER XXV

VAGINISMUS

VAGINISMUS means the painful spasm of the vagina due to local hyperaesthesia of the vaginal walls.

It may be superficial or deep according as the seat is at the entrance of the vagina, or probaly in the bulbo-cavernous muscle, or in the levator—ani muscle.

Various names have been given to this condition according to the underlying causing factor : for example—

1. Mental vaginismus.
2. Perineal vaginismus.
3. Posterior vaginismus.
4. Vulvar vaginismus.

1. Mental Vaginismus :—In this condition, there is complete aversion to sexual performance on the part of the woman, alongwith the contraction of the vaginal and vulval muscles when the act is attempted.

2. Perineal Vaginismus :—This condition is due to the spasm of perineal muscles.

3. Posterior Vaginismus :—It is caused by the spasm of the levatorani muscles.

4. Vulvar Vaginismus- :It is that from of vaginismus which is caused by the spasm of the constrictor viginal muscle.

Treatment

1. Find out the underlying cause and treat accordingly.

   In case of mental causation, reassurance of the patient is very essential.

2. *Homoeopathic remedies* :

   The following remedies may be given with good results according to the symptomatology of the case :—

   Cactus G., Plumbum Met., Bell., Cauloph, Cimicif; Cocculus, Coffea, Gels; Ign., Nat. Mur., Mag. Phos, Murex, Platina, Thuja.

Arnica :—Vaginismus, after forced attempts at coition.

Belladonna :—Convulsive motion of the vaginal muscles. With dryness, heat and burning in the vagina, and dragging in the loins; cutting pain from hip to hip. Worse, touch, jar and lying down. Rush of blood to the head and face; so the face looks red and eyes blood-shot. Sudden acute attack of the disease, with contraction of the sphincter muscle; hence coition is very painful.

Cactus G. :—Vaginismus, with constriction of the muscular fibres, as of an iron band. Constriction in the uterine region and ovaries. Dysmenorrhoea with pulsating pains in the uterus and ovaries. Menses are early, dark and pitch-like; they stop on lying down. The complaints are generally attanded by heart symptoms. The patient is sad and melancholic; has fear of death; is anxious; and screams with pain. Merely touching the parts causes constriction of the vagina, and so, prevents coition.

Caulophyllum :—Vaginismus, with spasmodic and severe pains, which fly in all directions. Affection, occuring after labour. Has needle like pains in the cervix. Often attended by rheumatism of the small joints.

Cimicifuga :—This remedy is especially useful in the rheumatic and nervous patients, with overian irritation, uterine cramps and heavy limbs. Vaginismus, with crampy pains; pains are as like electric shocks; pain across the pelvis from hip to hip. She has great depression with dreams of impending evil. Has uneasy, restless feeling and aching in the limbs and muscular soreness. Pain in lumbar and sacral regions, down the things and through hips.

Cocculus :—Spasmodic pains. Dysmenorrhoea, with profuse derk menses. Very weakening leucorrhoea, that she can hardly speak. It is especially suitable in cases of light-haired ladies, causing much nausea and backache, unmarried and childness women, sensitive and romantic girls. The patient feels worse when riding in a carriage. She is capricious, heavy and stupid, and has profound sadness; time passes too quickly.

Coffea :—Vulva and vagina hypersensitive; voluptuous itching. Vaginismus : from sudden emotions; with great nervous excitability and intolerance of pain. Extreme sensitiveness is the keynote for this remedy. It is especially suited to tall, thin, stooping patients, with dark complexion and choleric and sanguine, temperament.

Gelsemium :—Vaginismus, Dysmenorrhoea, with scanty flow of menses; the pain extends to the back and hips; aphonia and sore throat during menses. There is a sensation as if the uterus were squeezed. With dull aching in lumbar and sacral regions, passing upward. Dizziness, dullness drowsiness and trembling, are generally present in almost all the complaints. Muscular weakness with complete relaxation and prostration. Worse, cold and dampness. Headache preceded by blindness, better by profuse urination.

Ignatia :—The affection due to nervous and hysterical factors; it is especially adapted to the women who are sensitive, of easily excited nature, dark, of mild disposition, quick to perceive and rapid in execution. Exaggeration of the acuteness of symtoms. The patient is melancholic, sad, tearful and silently brooding. Sighing and, sobbing at small intervals is characteristic. The patient poses to be sick, she is not actually sick. Feeling of a lump in throat that cannot be swallowed; globus-hystericus. Has sinking in the stomach, which is relieved by takin a deep breath.

Lycopodium .—Dryness of vagina, with pain during and after coition.

Mag. Phos :—Vaginismus; spasmodic contractions of the muscles of the vagina; ovarian neuralgia and swelling of the external genitals accompany. Painful menses, of the membranous type. She feels better by the external application of heat. Especially suited to tired languid and exhausted patients.

Murex:-This remedy is particularly adapted to the nervous, lively and affectionate women; the patient is very weak and run down; she has great sadness, anxiety and fear. The parts are very sensitive; least contact causes great sexual excitement. Pain from right side of the uterus going to right or left breast.

Natrum Mur :—The vagina is dry with oedema; so it causes painful contractions of the vagina at coition. Great weakness and weariness, mostly felt in the morning in bed. Consolation aggravates. Aversion to coition. Chronic affection in anaemic women.

Platina :—The parts are hypersensitive, with hysterical spasms; pains increase and decrease gradually. Nymphomania. Excessive sexual development; vaginismus; and pruritus vulva. Has superiority complex; contempt for others. Cramp-like squeezing pain in the vagina.

Plumbum Met :—Vaginismus with emaciation and constipation; induration of mammary glands; vulva and vagina hypersensitive. Disposition to yawn and stretch. The patient is full of mental depression and has a fear of being murdered.

Thuja :—History of gonorrhoea may be traced. The vagina is very sensitive; any attempt at coition causes contraction of the muscles, making the act painful and difficult. Warty growths on the vulva and perineum. Profuse leucorrhoea, which is thick and greenish. Rapid exhaustion and emaciation. Hydrogenoid constitution; hence, worse by cold damp air. The patient has fixed ideas; as if a strange person is by her side; as if something alive in the abdomen.

— —

CHAPTER XXVI

PATHOLOGICAL VAGINAL DISCHARGES

Not only leucorrhoea, blood, pus, urine and sometimes faecal matter also, are included under this heading.

Aetiology

1. These discharges may come from vagina, cervix, uterus, tubes, bladder, rectum, ureters, peritoneal cavity and cellular tissues.
2. They may be gonococcal, streptococcal, staphylococcal, pneumococcal, B. Coli and so on.
3. Vaginal bacilli (duoderlane) are absent in these discharges and they are usually alkaline.
4. They may be due to Trichomonas vaginalis (thread worms enter through rectum).
5. They may be non-infective and due to general causes, like, anaemia.
6. They may be due to chronic constipation.
7. Sometimes leucorrhoea is due to persistent hard hymen.

Leucorrhoea or white discharge may be due to :—

1. Normal excess per and post menstrual congestion.
2. Congestion caused by pregnancy.
3. Anaemia and bad health.
4. Chronic inflammation of vagina.

Ropy or Mucoid Discharge :—This may be due to endocervicitis.

Purulent Discharge :—It may be due to :

1. Acute or chronic vaginitis.
2. Pelvic abscess draining through vagina
3. Senile-endometritis,

4. Pyometra, or
5. Chronic gonorrhoea.

Offensive Discharge :—This may be due to :

1. Ulcerated malignant tumour, like cancer of cervix.
2. Neglected pessary.
3. Sapraemia (when dead tissue is coming out of the uterus).
4. Sloughing submucous fibroids.
5. Incomplete abortion.

Watery Discharge :—The reasons may be :

1. Ruptured vaginal cysts.
2. Intermitent hydrosalpinx
3. Tubal cancer.
4. Hyperplastic endometritis.

Bloody Discharge :—This may occur due to the following reasons :

1. Injury.
2. Ulceration from retained pessary in procedentia.
3. Malignant tumours of uterus, cervix and vagina.
4. Polypi.
5. Abortion.
6. Ectopic gestation.
7. Carunclae.

Urinary Discharge :—It may come from the bladder or ureters in vesico-vaginal fistula.

Faecal Discharge :—It comes from the recto-vaginal fistula.

Treatment

Treatment depends upon the cause, the type of discharge and age of the patient.

Routine douching with antiseptics is not only useless, but at times, harmful. If douche is absolutely necessary, only boiled water or distilled water should be used.

Some patients will get well when their constipation is properly treated.

If hymen is very tight, perinectomy is advised.

Homoeopathic remedies :

Alumina, Calc. Carb., Hydras., Puls., Thuja, Sulphur, and any other remedy under the chapter Leucorrhoea, of course according to symptoms.

THERAPEUTIC HINTS

Alumina :—Leucorrhoea acrid, profuse, transparent and ropy, with burning, and going upto the heels ; worse during day and after menses ; and relieved by washing with cold water. The patient has abnormal cravings, like chalk, charcoal, dry food, tea grounds, etc. Potatoes do not agree.

Calcarea Carb. :—Leucorrhoea is milky; burning and itching of parts before and after menses and in little girls; milk too abundant in the breasts, does not agree to the child; much sweat about external genitals ; the menses are early, profuse and last long, with toothache, vertigo and cold, damp feet. In fact, flabby patients, who have craving for indigestible things, like chalk, coal, pencils, etc.

Hydrastis :—Leucorrhoea acrid and corroding, shreddy and tenacious ; worse after menses. Pruritus vulva, with leucorrhoea. There is dull, heavy dragging pain and stiffness, particularly across the lumber region ; so she must use her arms in raising herself from the seat. It is especially suitable in old, easily tired people, cachetic individuals ; with great debility.

Medorrhinum :—The menses are offensive, profuse, dark and clotted; stains are difficult to was out, passes urine frequently at that time. Leucorrhoea is thin, acrid, and excoriating and of fishy-odour. With a history of sycosis.

Pulsatilla :—Leucorrhoea acrid, burning and creamy; with pain in back and tired feeling. All other symptoms of Pulsatilla are present.

Sulphur :—Leucorrhoea, burning and excoriating ; vagina burns; and the pudenda itches. Flushes of heat; dry and hard skin; redness of orifices ; and sinking feeling at the stomach at 11 A.M.

Thuja :—Profuse leucorrhoea, think and greenish. Vagina is very sensitive. Warty growths on the vulva and perineum. Profuse perspiration before menses, especially on covered parts. A great anti-sycotic remedy. Hydrogenoid constitution.

Other remedies :—The remedies discussed under the chapter on **Leucorrhoea** should also be consulted.

—/—

CHAPTER XXVII

DISEASES OF THE CERVIX

ACUTE ENDOCERVICITIS

As the cervix is situated away from the exterior, it is not liable to infection quickly. But at the same time, it is abundantly supplied with blood. So, once it gets infected, it is very difficult to cope with the infection.

ACUTE ENDOCERVICITIS :—means an acute inflammation of the mucous membrane lining the canal of the cervix uteri.

Laceraction of the cervix at childbirth predisposes to cervical infection.

Aetiology

1. Laceration of the cervix, either due to childbirth or any operative interference.

2. Gonococcus and all other pyogenic bacteria.

Signs and Symptoms

1. Muco-purulent discharge from the vagina due to pyogenic infection.

2. Cervix inflamed, soft and tender.

3. On examination : Cervix is found red; there is erosion and ulceration over the cervix; and the external os will be found red and inflamed.

4. Alongwith these symptoms certain constitutional symptoms are also present; such as,

(i) rise of temperature,

(ii) headache, etc.

Treatment

1. Bed rest is compulsory, especially when the condition is acute.

2. Modern treatment is the antibiotic treatment : during culture, sulpha drugs are used.

3. *Homoepathic remedies* :

Bell., Ars., Hepar sulph., Hydras., Merc. Sol., Nit. ac., Puls., Thuja and Medo. depending upon the indications of each drug.

CHAPTER XXVIII

CHRONIC ENDOCERVICITIS

CHRONIC ENDOCERVICITIS means the chronic and a low grade inflammation of the mucous membrane of the cervical canal.

Aetiology

1. Sequela of the acute endocervicitis.

2. Sepsis after Labour or abortion, especially the criminal abortion.

3. Urinary infections extending to cervix through the vaginal canal.

4. Excessive production of oestrin, i.e., hyperplasia of epithelial lining causing a non-inflammatory type of chronic endocervicitis.

Sings and Symptoms

In non-inflammatory type of chornic endocervicitis, the symptoms would be :

1. Locorrhoeal discharge.
2. Cervix found enlarged.
3. Distended follicles erosions: the condition is known as ECTROPION—meaning abortion of the lips of cervix.

Treatment

1. Destroy the overgrowth by cauterization or diathermy. But, it is only a palliative treatment.

2. Then, treat the patient constitutionally with appropriate *homoeopathic drugs* :—

Ars., Hepar Sulph., Medo., Puls., Conium, Carbo an., Sulph. ac., etc.

CHAPTER XXIX

EROSION OF CERVIX

Erosion of Cervix —is the desquamation of the epithelium on the vaginal surface adjacent to the external os. In the erosion, a single layer of columnar epithelium is involved under which are aggregations of inflammatory cells. This erosion has a tendency to heal; but when it extends, it becomes an ulcer.

Aetiology

1. Prolonged use of pessaire and chemical contraceptives.
2. Infection of the cervix, especially,
   (i) Gonococcal infection, and
   (ii) Puerperal, i.e., post-delivery infection.
3. Excessive secretion of oestrin.
4. Congenital erosion where the patches of columnar epithelium remain adhered to the cervix.
5. Excessive alkalinity of the vaginal secretion.

Signs and Symptoms :

1. Lecuorrhoeal discharge, yellowish white in colour and containing desquamated vaginal epithelial cells.
2. If it is septic, the discharge is mucopurulent and offensive.
3. Lecorrhoea profuse, before and after the menses.
4. Pain in the lower abdomen before and during menses.
5. Infection may spread to the bladder, and so there may be frequency of micturition or dysuria.
6. Menorrhagia.
7. This may result into chronic ill-health and rheumatoid arthritis.

8. On examination :
   (i) Red patches can be seen on the cervix or in the neighbourhood of external os.
   (ii) There is redness and swelling of the cervical mucosa.
   (iii) Feeling of the part is velvet-like.
   (iv) There may be slight bleeding on touch.
   (v) External os is soft and patulous.
   (vi) Mucous polypi are often seen attached to the margin of external os.
   (vii) The cervix is found thickened.
   (viii) There is a feeling of pain on moving the cervix.

The infection may spread to the pelvis causing inflammation of the pelvic cellular tissues.

Differential Dignosis

Erosion in an aged woman must be differentially diagnosed from carcinoma of the cervix.

	Carcinoma	*Erosion*
1.	There will be bleeding on touch, palpation or intercourse.	No bleeding on touch or intercourse.
2.	The lesion is hard and the edges are slightly raised.	The lesion is not hard but soft and not raised.

When are in doubt, send the patient for biopsy to the pathologist to know whether cancerous cells are present or not.

Treatment

1. Cauterization and diathermy.
2. In cases who resist cauterization, amputation of the cervix is advised.
3. Frequent douches with hydrastis lotion, Echinacea lotion are very important in the treatment of cervical erosion.

4. Then, indicated *homoeopathic remedies* :

Ars., Arg. Nit., Aur. Mur. Nat., Carbolic Acid, Carbo-An., Fl. Ac., Hydras., Kreosote, Merc., Sulph., Thuja, Ustilago, Vespa, Kali Bich., and Nat. Mur.

THERAPEUTIC HINTS

Argentum Nitricum :—Head remedy. Bleeding accompanied with prolapse. Discharge is albuminous.

Argentum Met :—May be used if the above remedy fails. Symptoms are similar but tending to malignancy.

Kreosote :—Foetid acrid discharge. Ulceration on the cervix; bleeds easily.

Sulphuric Acid :—Erosion in the aged patients.

Arsenic :—Foetid acrid discharge with ulceration.

Thuja :—Faulty menses which are very irregular, sometimes appearing at long intervals with profuse discharge but bleeding all along.

Conium :—If there is stony hardness.

Carbolic Acid :—Erosion of cervix with foetid, acrid discharge. Pain in left ovary, worse walking in open air. Agonizing backache across the loins, with dragging upon the thighs.

Carbo Animalis :—Cancer of cervix, with induration and burning pains with thin offensive discharge from the vagina.

For other remedies, kindly consult the therapeutic hints under the Chapters "Diseases of the Uterus" and "Tumours of the uterus."

——

CHAPTER XXX

DISEASES OF THE UTERUS

Acute Endometritis

ACUTE ENDOMETRITIS is the acute inflammation of mucous of the uterus which is known as the endometrium.

Aetilogy

1. Puerperal sepsis, i.e. infection after delivery.
2. Criminal interference at abortion.
3. Organisms responsible are all the pyogenic bacteria; such as—Streptococci, Staphylococci, Haemoytica pyogenia, B. Coli, B. Walchi., etc.

Sings and Symptoms

1. Rise of temperature.
2. Rise of pulse rate, out of proportion to temperature.
3. Malaise.
4. Abdominal pain.
5. Sometimes, feeling of chilliness and rigor is prominently present.
6. The uterus is found to be tender on palpation.
7. In puerperal cases :

   The uterus is enlarged and the lochia will be excessive and offensive.
8. In non-puerperal cases :

   Profuse menorrhagia and blood stained discharge is the important phenomenon.

Complication

1. **General septicaemia** may occur if the infection is not stopped and when it enters the blood stream. It is a serious

complication in the untreated and maltreated cases, and if proper attention is not given, grave results may follow.

2. **Thrombophlebitis :** It means the development of venous thrombi in the presence of inflammatory changes in the vessel wall.

3. **Salpingitis :** It is the inflammation of the fallopian tubes. The genital tract is a continuous passage from below upwards. So, the infection in the uterus may extend upwards causing salpingitis.

4. **Pelvic peritonitis :** As the genital tract is a continuous passage extending from the vulva to the peritoneum through the fimbriae, the infection can travel up to the peritoneum of the pelvic region causing pelvic-peritonitis and even general peritonitis, of course, in unfavourable cases.

5. **Pelvic cellulitis :** It is also called parametritis. It means a diffuse inflammatory process within the solid tissues of the pelvis characterized by oedema, redness, pain and interference with function.

Prognosis

Prognosis is not bad if detected and treated early, with suitable homoeopathic remedies when the complications have not set in.

Treatment

1. Complete bed rest is necessary as the condition is and acute one.

2. Diet regimen : fluid and nutritious diet.

3. Then, the ***homoeopathic remedies*** :

Ars., Rhus Tox. Bell., Pyrogen, Baptisia. Lach., Aco., Bry., Ferrum-Phos., Hepar Sulp., Silicea, Merc. Sol., Sulph.

——

CHAPTER XXXI

CHRONIC ENDOMETRITIS

CHRONIC ENDOMETRITIS means the chronic inflammation of the endometrial lining of the uterus, which may develop due to a number of causes. The condition, here, is not an acute one, but at the same time, the symptoms do not disappear at all at any time and there is a sort of low grade infection causing a continuous inflammatory process in the endometrium.

Aetiology

1. As a sequela of acute endometritis.
2. Hormonal imbalances.
3. Pyometra or infected polypus, etc.
4. I. U. C. D.
5. Tuberculosis.
6. Conococcal infection.

1. As a Sequela of Acute Endometritis :— Actually it is a rare condition As, with every menstrual cycle there is the shedding off of the endometrium and also the new growth of the endometrium, so it is not infected usually; but, if some matter remains after the acute condition, chronic endometritis may follow.

2. Hormonal Imbalances:— If there is excess of oestrin secretion, it will cause hypertrophy and thickening of the endometrium, so the infection may occur. Similarly, if there is lack of oestrin, it will cause thinning of the endometrium. Natural barriers to infection are also affected when there is lack of glycogen and acidity in the vaginal secretions ; so, the chances of infection ascending to the uterus are more.

3. Pyometra or Infected Polypus :— Pyometra means the formation and collection of pus in the uterus. Due to an obstruction in the drainage of pus and discharge from the uterus, the pus will go on collecting causing it to bulge out. Obstruction is due to a tumour or the collection of pus itself.

4. I. U. C. D. :—It stands for the intrauterine contraceptive devices; e. g., loop. Constant and prolonged use of these intra-uterine devices may also cause inflammation of the endometrium due to constant and prolonged irritation thus caused.

5. Tuberculosis :—This infection is very rare in the involvement of the uterus. However, tubercular salpingitis is more common.

6. Conococcal Infection :—Gonorrhoea, being the main infection of the genital tract, cannot be ruled out in the causation of the chronic inflammation of the endometrium.

Signs And Symptoms

1. It mainly occurs in the parous, sterile and virgin women, between the age of puberty and menopause.
2. Lecorrhoea, due to infection of the cervix.
3. Menorrhagia : the periods are prolonged, but, usually there is no severe flooding.
4. Dysmenorrhoea, common in multipara, of course.
5. Pain in the pelvis between the periods.
6. Sterility is common. But if pregnancy occurs, it generally aborts quickly.
7. Purulent discharge.
8. Cervical erosion may be present.
9. The uterus is somewhat enlarged.

Investigations

Exclude cancer by curettage and biopsy.

Treatment

Certain points are to be kept in mind while treating such case :

1. Treat the cause first.
2. Curetting of the uterus, generally helps in correcting the condition.
3. Then, the suitable *homoeopathic remedies* :

Aur. Met., Aur. Mur. Nat., Borax, Calc. Carb., Cimicifuga, Graph., Hydrastis, Helonias, Mag. Mur., Puls., Sepia, Sulphur, Lach., etc.

CHAPTER XXXII

SENILE ENDOMETRITIS

Inflammation of the endometrial lining of the uterus occuring in old age is known as SENILE ENDOMETRITIS.

Aetiology

The cause, here, is the post-menopausal atrophy causing a low grade infection by the vaginal organisms.

As there is a decrease in the secretion of oestrin, there is no growth of the endometrium and thus there is atrophy. The vaginal acidity decreases, so, the infection occurs first in the vagina and then it goes to the uterus.

Primary condition, in old age, is the atrophy and then the infection takes place causing senile endometritis.

Sings and Symptcms

1. Offensive discharge ; it may be blood stained also.
2. Uterus is soft and small ; but enlarged, if pyometra is present.

Post-menopausal age is more prone to cancer formation ; so, get the biopsy done to exclude the possibility of cancer. If, that is not present, then we can be sure of senile endometritis.

Diagnosis

The diagnosis can be made by differentiating the condition from cancer by getting the biopsy done.

Treatment

1. Eradicate infection by douching with antiseptics and drugs.
2. Give oestrin-preparations, like Stilboestrol (oestrin+a little progesterone).
3. Then, treat with homoeopathic medicines, especially the constitutional *remedies* :

Phos., Lach., Sabina, Hama., Bell., China, Ustilago, Lil. Tig., Plus., Sulphur, etc.

CHAPTER XXXIII

DISEASES OF THE FALIOPIAN TUBES

ACUTE SALPINGITIS

ACUTE SALPINGITIS means an inflammation of the fallopian tubes occuring on account of a number of causes. It may involve both the sides or only one side at the some time.

Aetiology

1. Ascending infection from the vagina or cervix..
2. Direct infection from adjacent visceras.
3. Infection through the blood stream.
4. Infection through the abdominal opening. Usually both the tubes are affected, but if only one tube is involved. it soon becomes a bilateral condition.

The ovaries are also infected invariably causing salpingo-oophoritis.

Mode of Infection :

All the 4 modes of infection are there :

1. **Ascending Infection from Vagina or Cervix :** Ascending infection occurs due to any infection of the genital tract. The organisms responsible for the infection are Gonococci, Streptococci and Staphylococci.

2. **Direct Infection from Adjacent Viscera :** If the appendix is inflammed, the infection may travel to the fallopian tube on the right side first, then extending the infection to the other tube soon after. The organisms responsible mostly are B. Coli and Streptococcus faecalis.

3. **Infection through blood Stream :** Infection through the blood stream may come from the distant places ; such as, tonsillitis ; but it is a rare condition. Tuberculosis is, however, more common.

4. Infection through Abdominal Opening : Infection may also come from the abdominal opening, such as pèritonitis.

Sings and Symptoms

1. History of recent delivery, abortion or operation on the cervix may be available.
2. Gonorrhoeal infection of the husband of wife may be traced.
3. Fever with rigor, it being the pyogenic infection.
4. Pain in the lower abdomen inguinal region.
5. Vomiting may be present, especially in the beginning, due to the toxaemic state of the blood.
6. Purulent vaginal discharge—leucorrhoea :

   (Purulent discharge means the infection is present. And, non-purulent discharge is the transudation from passive congestion).
7. Irregular, heavy and profuse menses (the discharge is mucoid or muco-purulent).
8. Tenderness and rigidity over the lower abdomen at tubal points.
9. On P.V. examination, i.e., vaginal examination at a later stage, the tubes can be felt in the lateral fornices as thick masses, i.e., cord like structures and inflamed.
10. If the pelvic abscess has formed, a fluctuating tender bulge can be felt in ehe posterior fornix.

Invastigations

1. **T.L.C.** It will show leucocytosis. In inflammations and infections, leucocytosis is found, because it is a defensive mechanism of the body against the invading organisms.

2. **Vaginal Swab Tests :** For culture and sensitivity.

Diagnosis

The disgnosis is confirmed by the following points :—

1. Careful history :

   History of genorrhoea of the male or female is often present.

2. Presence of vaginal discharges or even bleeding.
3. Diffuse tenderness and rigidity.

   Salpingitis of even one side may cause tenderness and rigidity of the other side also.

4. Tenderness at a difinite point (as is in appendicitis, i.e., at the Mcburhy's point) is not there.
5. Movement of the cervix will cause lot of pain.
6. Bimanual examination :

   One will find the tenderness just above the pubis may be in one or the other side.

7. Through laparotomy :

   Here, the surgeon comes to help : he advises immediate, laparotomy. If the appendix is found to be inflamed it is removed ; but the tubes are not removed, rather a drain is provided to relieve the tension and distension.

Differential Diagnosis :

Salpingitis should be differentially diagnosed from the following conditions :

1. Acute appendicitis.
2. Rupture of tubal-gestation.
3. Pyelitis.

1. Acute Appendicitis : In appendicitis, vomiting is important and the pain is localized at the Mcburny's point. It is not an emergency condition in the beginning when there is no abscess ; but, it may rupture and cause peritonitis ; that is, it becomes an emergency at a later stage.

2. **Rupture of Tubal Gestation :** When there is rupture of ectopic pregnancy, it is a serious condition and needs surgery immediately. Not the shock-symptoms, such as, pallor, breathlessness, sweating, restlessness, fall in temperature, fall in the blood pressure air and hunger.

As the pain is important in all the three conditions, in the case of rupture there will be extreme tenderness and rigidity of the abdomen : if the pain is in the inguinal region, try to find out the emergency condition.

3. **Pyelitis :** Pyelitis means inflammation of the pelvis of the kidney. In this condition, the pain is felt in the lumbar region primarily ; it may, however, travel to the front. Order for the urine examination; it will show albumen and pus cells.

Treatment :

1. Rest in bed, as in all cases of infection.
2. Plenty of alkaline fluids : barley water is alkaline ; soda-water or soda bicarb, with water is alkaline.
3. Modern antibiotics are started immediately after the infection, e.g., penicillin, streptomycin, chloromycetin, and then send to the laboratory for culture and sensitivity tests.
4. Analgesics and sedatives for pain, such as, novalgin, etc.
5. Laxatives for bowel movements, if required ; but enema must be avoided.
6. No vaginal interference, such as douching, etc.
7. Dry heat on the abdomen and hot fomentation for allaying the pain and inflammation. If pelvic abscess forms and it points through the posterior fornix, then do drainage through posterior colpotomy, i.e., incision through the vaginal fornix.
8. After all, the appropriate homoeopathic drugs among the acute group :

Aco., Bell., Apis, Ars., Bry., Canth., Hepar Sulph., Merc., Sulphur, Silicea, Puls., etc.

——

CHAPTER XXXIV

CHRONIC SALPINGITIS

CHRONIC SALPINGITIS is the chronic inflammation of the fallopian tubes; and it is invariably always due to the acute condition mentioned earlier.

Signs and Symptoms

1. Vague pain in the lower abdomen, because of certain amount of chronic infection present in the body—pelvis.
2. Backache: due to the presence of chronic cellular tissue infection in the body.
3. Painful and profuse menstruation.
4. Leucorrhoea.
5. Dyspareunia, i.e. pain during intercourse.
6. General weakness.
7. Anaemia.
8. Recurrent attacks of fever with pelvic pain, because some infection is remaining.
9. **On abdominal examination** :—Firm cystic masses felt over the inguinal ligaments—½″ above the ligaments where the tubes are lying : they are placed parallel to the ligaments on both sides.

   Cystic swelling coatains fluid and the solid swelling is solid. Similarly, cystic tumours contain fluid, whether pus or simple.

   In flammatory condition, there is always hyperaemia, active or passive, because of the chronic inflammation and there is pus also.
10. **On P.V. examination** :—Thickness of cord-like structures felt on palpation in the two lateral fornices.

Treatment

There are two aspects of the treatment—Medical and Surgical.

Certain important factors are to be kept in mind while treating a case of chronic salpingitis :—

1. Treat the infection first.
2. Try to improve the general health of the patient—with diet, drugs and exercise.
3. Dry hot for mentation for allaying the pains.

Surgical treatment :—Surgical treatment is given to those cases who form the adhesions there. It is only done in post—menopausal period.

Medicinal treatment :—After all this, come the appropriate homoeopathic remedies of chornic phase; e.g.,

Lach., Sepia, Thuja, Medo., Sulphur, etc.

And then, the constitutional drugs : e.g.,

Sil., Ferrup phos., Nat. Mur., Calc. Carb., Calc. Phos, and others according to the symptoms.

Acids are given in non-infective cases to induce more urination, so that the toxins are thrown out.

THERAPEUTIC HINTS

(Diseases of The Uterus And Faliopian Tubes)

Aesculus hipp. :—Pain in the small of the back and hip, with a lame feeling; the pain extends from the abdomen to the small of the back, which makes it almost impossible to get up and to walk after sitting; constipation and piles.

Aconite :—High fever; dry skin; intense thirst; great restlessness; fear of death, and predicting the hour of death.

Aletris farinosa :—In cases of debility from protracted illness, loss of fluids, defective nutrition, etc; great disposition to abortion.

Alumina :—Profuse, purulent, yellow, corroding discharge, worse before and after the menses; during the day only; vertigo, constipation.

Ambra Grisea :—Discharge only at night; thick mucus with stitches in the vagina before the discharge; pieces of bluish-white mucus.

Arsenic :—Burning pain; indescribable anguish and restlessness; sudden sinking of strength; burning thirst, drinks often, but little at a time; cold drinks make her worse; burning in the veins; aggravation about midnight.

Belladonna :—Violent pains by spells; clutching pains, as is fingers with nails were clawing the intestines together; meteorism, with eructations; great sensitiveness and heat in the abdomen; painful bearing down in the pelvis towards the genitals and the rectum, with constant, ineffectual desire for stool; suppression of the lochial or menstrual discharge, or else vitiated, foetid discharge. Congestion of the head, with delirium, redness of face, and throbing of the carotid arteries; drowsy dozing with startings, or drowsiness, with inability to go to sleep.

Bryonia :—Wants to lie perfectly still; the slightest motion causes pain; in the head splitting pain; in the bowels, limbs and body stitch-like pain; great dryness in the mouth, without thirst, or else great thirst, drinking tumbler after tumbler; perspiration in short spells, and only on single parts of the body; constipation.

Cālc carb :—Fat persons, and those whose menses are too profuse and return too soon ; they sweat easily about the head, and are troubled constantly with cold and damp feet Chronic infarction of the womb.

Cantharis :—Constant painful urging and tenesmus of the bladder; like-wise, in worst cases, when the patient lies unconscious with her arms stretched out along the side of her body, interrupted by sudden starting up, screaming, throwing about the arms and even convulsions; all signs of erosions and ulceration of internal organs.

Caulophyllum :—Insomnia; paraplegia; atony and relaxed condition of the uterus; hysterical spasms; irregular menstruation; excessive uterine haemorrhage.

Chamomilla :—Great agitation of the nervous system; she seems beside herself, with red face and heat all over ; she is ill-humored, and can scarcely restrain herself to treat people with civility; sometimes one cheek red and the other pale; after fits of passion.

Colocynth :—Colicky pains in the bowels, with deadly colour of the face and bending double; worse after eating or drinking; partial heat and partial coolness of the skin, with quick pulse, vomiting and diarrhoea; bitter taste in the mouth; after indigestion.

Conium :—Swelling of the breasts; stitches in the breast, mostly at night; induration of the cervix, with sharp pains in the part; acrid leucorrhoea; prolapus uteri.

Crocus:—Black stringy discharge; rolling and bounding in the abdomen, as from a foetus; stitching in the abdomen arresting respiration.

Gelsemium :—Hysteria; hyperaesthesia of a part of the body; tendency to hemiplegia, confusion of mind; sleeplessness; spasms; fever, without thirst, intermittent; nervous exhaustion.

Hyoscyamus :—Typhoid state; either complete apathy, or else great exciteability, spasms, jerkings, delirium, wild starting, throwing off bed clothes, leaving herself naked; bright red clots after child-birth.

Kreosote :—Putrid state of the womb after child-birth; confounding ideas; loss of memory; thinks herself well; discharge of dark offensive blood from the womb.

Lachesis :—Constantly lifting the bed clothes from the abdomen, on account of uneasy feeling caused by it; the pain in the uterus is relieved by a flow of blood for the time being, but recturns soon afterwards; in bad cases, unconsciousness, livid face, repeated shaking chills ; skin alternately burning hot and cold; abdomen distended; lochial discharge thin, ichorous; stool and urine suppressed.

Mercurius :—Inflammation of the genital organs and ulcers; moist, soft tongue, showing the imprints of the teeth, accompanied occasionally with great thirst; profuse sweat without relief; all worse at night.

Nux vomica :—After taking cold, or using various kinds of dugs; in chronic cases, with bearing down into the vagina and towards the os, sacrum; constant urging to urinate; constipation.

Phosphorus :—Fair graceful women; after frequent pregnancies; pyaemic state and inflammation of the veins.

Pulsatilla :—After getting the feet wet; frequent chilliness; thirstlessness; deficiency of milk; suppression of the lochial discharge; mild, tearful disposition.

Rhus tox :—Constant restless moving; can't lie still; dry tongue, with red tip; red rash on the breast; powerlessness of the lower limbs ; the lochial discharge turns bloody again ; typhoid symptoms.

Sabina :—In metritis haemorrhagica.

Secale cor :—Putrescence of the uterus; abdomen distended, not very painful; discharge from the vagina, brownish, offensive; ulcers on the external genitals discolored and repidly spreading ; burning hot fever ; interrupted by shaking chills; small, sometimes intermittent pulse; great anguish; pain in the pit of the stomach, vomiting decomposed matter; offensive diorrhoea; suppressed secretion of urine; the skin is covered with petechial and miliary eruptions, or shows discoloured, inflamed places, with a tendency to mortification; the patient lies either in quiet delirium, or grows wild with great anxiety and a constant desire to get out of bed.

Sepia :—Painful stiffness in the uterine region; bearing down; sense of weight in anus; sense of goneness in obdomen; yellowish spots on the face.

Sulphur :—Frequent weak, faint spells, especially before noon; bearing down, especially on standing; leucorrhoea; soreness of genitals.

Veratrum ablbum :—If commencing with violent fits of vomiting and diarrhoea; hot body; cold extremities and deadly pale face, covered with cold perspiration; delirium and great anxiety; suppressed lochial discharge; nymphomania.

Veratrum viride :—Congestion of pelvic organs, tenderness of uterus; fever; heat; restlessness; palpitation of heart; local or general hyperaesthesia.

CHAPTER XXXV

DISEASES OF THE OVARIES

OOPHORITIS

OOPHORITIS means inflammation of the ovary, which may be unilateral or bilateral at the same time.

It my be acute or chronic in occurance. In the acute form, the symptoms would be that of acute inflammation and in the chronic form, the symptoms would indicate a chronic and low grade infection.

Aetiology

1. **Secondary to salpingitis** :— Acute and chronic inflammatory diseases are invariably often associated with salpingitis.

2. **Metastatic from parotitis** :—Exact explanation for the relation between parotitis and oophoritis is of course, cannot be given ; but, it happens in certain girls and young women.

3. **Ovarian abscess** :— Abscess of the ovary may be due to salpingitis (in a majority of cases) and tuberculosis.

4. **Pelvic peritonitis**

5. **Pelvic cellulitis**

Signs and Symptoms

Girls and young women, occasionally, complain of pelvic pain during an attack of momps, i.e., parotitis. In a few cases of severe variety, on P. V. examination, the ovaries are found to be enlarged, tender and painful. As a rule, the ovaries are affected during the subsidence of parotitis.

After pelvic peritonitis and cellulitis, the superficial parts of the ovary are infiltrated and adhere to the surrounding tissues. And, as the inflammatory products get organised, the voary/ovaries become imbedded in the tissue almost as dense as that of cicatrix. In this way, peri-oophoritis occurs, which is often. a sequel to typhoid, fever rheumatism, the exanthemata and chronic alcoholism.

Complications

The most important results of peri-oophori'tis are :—

1. Dysmenorrhoea, and
2. Sterility.

Treatment

Treatment is, of course, symptomatic. In case of acute inflammation, the general and non-medicinal treatment is the same as in other acute conditions of the pelvis.

Homoeopathic remedies :

Acute inflammation :

Aco., pis, Bell., Bry., Canth., Cimicif. Colch., Ham., Hepar Sulph., Iod., Lach., Merc. C., Puls., Thuja, Ars., Palladium, Aurum, Lilium Tig., Staph., Zinc., Arg. Met., Naja, Colocynth and Podophyllum.

Chronic inflammation :

Conium, Iod., Thuja, Medo., Sepia, Graph., Platina, etc., according to symptoms.

THERAPEUTIC HINTS

Aconite :—Headache, backache, colic, fever, great restlessness and tossing about; after exposure to cold winds or a sudden fright during the monthly period, by which the flow ceases; painful urging to urinate and to evacuate the bowels.

Antim crud :— when menstruation has been checked by taking a bath ; nausea and vomiting, white tongue ; great thirst at night ; alternate costiveness and diarhoea.

Apis:— Active congestion of the right ovary going on to inflammation ; swelling, with soreness in the inguinal region, burning, and stinging pains and tumefaction ; form sexual intercourse during the monthly period. Incipient ovarian eysts, with numbness in the right side of the abdomen, extending into the thigh, or upwards to the ribs ; scanty urine, retarded stool ; cough, with soreness and tightness in the upper portion of the left chest.

Arsenic :—Drawing, stitching burning pain from the region of the ovary into the thigh; which feels numb and lame, worse from motion, bending or sitting bent; burning pain in the back while lying quietly upon it; the menses consist of a thin, whitish, badly-smelling discharge; pale, yellowish face; emaciation; febrile action; thirst, with drinking little at a time; restlessness. Pains are relieved by hot applications.

Belladonna :—Acute oophoritis, more so if the peritoneum is involved. Hard swelling of the ovary, with stitching, clutching and throbbing pains; worse on right side. Slightest jar and the patient is highly sensitive; with constant bearing down, as if everything would issue out; fever, with perspiration; glistening eyes; red face and delirium; after child-birth. Sudden appearance of symptoms with flushed face, throbbing headache and other peculiar symptoms of the remedy are also present.

Bryonia :—Stitching pain, worse from the slightest motion and contact; suppression of the menses, with bleeding from the nose; inclined to constipation.

Cantharis :—Stitches, arresting the breathing; or violent pinching pains, with bearing down towards the genitals; or great burning pain in the ovarian region; constant urging and straining to urinate, with painful discharge of but a few drops of urine, which sometimes is bloody; after suppressed gonorrhoea.

Colocynth :—Cramp-like pain in the left ovarian region, as though the part were squeezed in a vice; colicky pain all over the abdomen, which causes the patient to bend double; pain in the left foot; worse before menstruation, which is more profuse.

Conium :—Chronic cases; induration; lancinating pains; pain in the mammae before the menses, which are feeble; smarting, excoriating leucorrhoea; giddiness when turning in bed; intermitting flow of urine.

Hamamelis :—Oophoritis with ovarian neuralgia. Subacute form of gonorrhoeal oophoritis. After a blow, the ovary swollen, with a diffuse agonizing soreness over the whole abdomen; menses irregular, very painful, with exacerbation of all the sufferings at the approach of menses, retention of urine.

Hepar Sulph. :—When suppuration takes place, indicated by frequent chills.

Ignatia :—Disappointed love; constant running of thoughts in that direction ; sighing, despondency ; leucorrhoea, which passes off with labour-like pains.

Lachesis :—Left ovary ; tensive, pressing pains and stitches; inability to lie on the right side, on account of sensation as if something were rolling over to that side ; menses scanty, with labour-like pressure from the loins downward ; swelling of the ovary; suppuration and chronic enlargement of the ovary. Pains are relieved by a discharge from the uterus. Can bear nothing heavy on the region of the ovary.

Mercurius :—Stitching, pressing pains in the lower region of the abdomen, left side ; upper portion of the abdomen distended ; stool with great tenesmus, constant urging to urinate, with scanty emission of a thick, brown-red urine, cousing burning in the urethra ; perspiration without relief ; great weakness and emaciation; nightly aggravation and restlessness ; menses suppressed.

Nux vomica :—After previous use of different allopathic drugs.

Platina :—Ovaries sensitive, burning pains in them, bearing down, chronic ovarian irritation. Excessive sexual desire, from an incessant tickling within the genitals; painful pressing towards the genital organs, as if the menses would make their appearance ; profuse of suppressed menses, with palpitation of the heart, headache, restlessness and weeping; haughtiness ; nymphomania. Much ovarian induration is present.

Pulsatilla :—After getting the feet wet; suppression of the menses, with nausea, coldness of the body, chilliness and trembling of the feet ; pressure on bladder and rectum ; thirstlessness, weeping meek disposition.

Rhus tox :—After getting wet, straining or lifting.

Zincum :—Boring pain in left ovary, relieved by pressure and during the menstrual flow; fidgety feet.

Merc Cor. :—Ovarian neuralgia ; with peritoneal complications.

Bovista :—Ovarian tumours.

Palladium :—Swelling and induration of right ovary. It lacks the mental symptoms of platina, such as mental egotism and excitement.

Lilium Tig. :—Ovarian neuralgias. Burning pains from ovary up into abdomen and down into thighs, shooting pain from left ovary across the pubes, or upto the mammary gland.

Staphisagria :—Very useful in ovarian irritation in nervous irritable women. Hypochondriacal moods.

Graphites :—Swelling and induration of left ovary ; also pains in right ovarian region with delayed scanty menses.

Argentum Met. :—Bruised pain in left ovary, and sensation as if the ovary were growing large.

Naja :—Violent crampy pain in left ovary. Useful in obscure ovarian pains not inflammatory in nature.

Iodine :—Congestion or dropsy or right ovary. Dwindling of mammae ; dull pressing, wedgelike pain, extending from right ovary to uterus like a plug, worse during menstruation.

Thuja :—Left sided cophoritis, with a history of venereal infection. Grumbling pains in the ovaries all the time, with mental irritability.

Podophyllum :—Pain in the right ovary, running down the thigh of that side. Numbness may also be present.

——

CHAPTER XXXVI

DISEASES OF THE PELVIC PERITONEUM

ACUTE PELVIC PERITONITIS

In some books, especially the old ones, it is written Perimetritis for Peritonitis, and Parametritis for Cellulitis.

ACUTE PELVIC PERITONITIS is the acute inflammation of the pelvic-peritoneum.

Aetiology

1. Puerpenal sepsis, e.g., endometritis :
   Sepsis occuring at the site from where the placenta is removed.
2. Abortion, especially the septic abortion.
3. Salpingitis.
4. Appendicitis.
5. Infective ovarian cysts.
6. Post-operational infection.
7. Organisms responsible are :
   Gonococci, Tubercle bacilli or other pyogenic bacteria.

Signs and Symptoms

1. History of abortion, delivery, tuberculosis or gonorrhoea.
2. Sudden rise of temperature with rigor and vomiting and tachycardia.
3. Acute pain in the lower abdomen, because the posibility of peritoneal involvement is there.

   In acute abdomens, the mortality rate is about 10% and in about 3-4 hours, it may rise to 50-60% if not cared for properly.
4. Rigidity and tenderness of the lower abdomen. When deeper tissues are involved, then rigidity or tenderness may be absent altogether.

5. On P.V. examination :

   Fornices are tender and painful and if pelvic abscess forms in the pouch of Doughlas, fluctuating tender swelling or mass is present in the pouch.

Prognosis

Prognosis is good if treated early as we shall check the spread of infection by early treatment.

Complications

If not treated properly and early, the infection may travel further causing :—

(i) General peritonitis.

(ii) Abscess formation in the pouch of Doughlas ; and thereafter.

(iii) Pelvic adhesions :

When these adhesions are formed, these can be corrected by surgical interference only.

(iv) Sterility :

If it is due to the formation of adhesions, it is not curable by drugs.

Treatment

1. Rest in bed, this being an acute condition.
2. Light, but nutritous diet.
3. Hot fomentation to allay the pains.
4. Artibiotics and sedatives.
5. Alkaline mixtures, and
6. Then, homoeopathic drugs :
   Aco., Bell., Bry., Merc. Sol, Lach., Ars. Iod., Ars. Alb., etc., etc.

If pelvic abscess forms in the pouch of Doughlas, then drainage is to be provided by posterior colpotomy.

THERAPEUTIC HINTS

Aconite :—Hot dry skin ; quick, hard, small pulse ; high inflammatory fever; mouth and tongue dry ; great thirst; bitter taste; vomiting; no stool; urine scanty; red and hot; lower extremities cool; short, quick breathing; very restless; anxious expression in the face; burning, cutting, darting pain in the bowels, worse from slightest pressure, motion and lying on the right side; abdomen hot to the touch. After taking cold, drinking cold water when being heated.

Apis :—Burning, stinging pain in the bowels, very sore to the touch; when exudation has taken place; urine scanty, dark; oedematous swelling of the feet; burning, stinging in the region of the ovaries; metritis.

Arnica :—After contusion; after an injury at the time of internal examination or a surgical operation.

Arsenic :—Later, when there is a sudden sinking of strength, cold, clammy perspiration, anxious, internal restlessness, insatiable thirst with drinking but little at a time; constant vomiting; burning in the bowels; all worse in the middle of the night.

Arsenic Iodide :—It is indicated by a profound prostration, rapid, irritable pulse, recurring fever and sweats, emaciation; tendency to diarrhoea. Emaciation notwithstanding good appetite. Amenorrhoea with anaemic palpitation and dyspnoea. Under this remedy, the discharges are acrid and burning. Diarrhoea thin, watery, acrid, corroding the anus. The patient has intense thirst; but the water is immediately ejected. Drenching night sweats. She is chilly, cannot endure cold.

Belladonna :—After Aconite, great congestion to the head; strongly pulsating carotid arteries; light and noise unbearable; colicky pain in the bowels; painful retching and vomiting, worse from motion and contact; great anxiety and dyspnoea. Especially when in complication with metrities or perityphlities.

Bryonia :—Stitching pain or pressing, lancinating in the bowels, worse from slightest motion; when exudation has taken place; tongue white and dry; great thirst; bowels constipated; the patient lies perfectly still, does not want to move. Especially in complication with diaphragmitis.

Calcarea Carb :—When about the seventh day a red rash appears ; also when the pain is alleviated by cold watrə applications, so that the patient wants them renewed constantly. Abdominal tuberculosis.

Cantharis :—Abdomen burning hot; tympanitic distension in its upper region; lower portion yields a dull sound; bloody, slimy stools; painful, extorting cries; tenesmus of the bladder; strangury; great anguish and restlessness; distressed face; sunken features; cold extremities. Especially when the serous covering of the bladder is the seat of inflammation.

Carbo Veg. :—Excessive tympanitis with paralysis of the bowels.

Lachesis :—Abdomen hot and sensitive to touch; painful stiffness from the loins down into the thighs: scanty; turbid urine with reddish sediment; strangury; constipation: necessity of laying on the back with drawn up knees. Especially in complication with typhlitis.

Lycopodium :–In complication with diaphrgmitis or hepatitis; when lying on the left side, a feeling as if a hard body were rolling from the navel to that side; or when after three or four days the face assumes a yellowish colour; troublesome flatulence and constipation; sleeplessness and constant distress.

Mercurius :—At a later period, if the exuded fluid becomes purulent, with frequent starts; creeping chills; perspiration without relief; pale, wretched complexion, foul smell from the mouth; vomiting of slime and slimy stools, with straining; oedematous swelling of the feat; great weakness and emaciation. Especially when in complication with typhlitis and the formation of abscesses.

Nitrum —Stitching and sticking pains; predominating coldness of the lower extremities; kind of numb and stiff feeling in the affected parts, as if they were made of wood.

Nux Vomica :—Belching, vomiting and constant pressure upon the rectum, as if urging to stool.

Opium :—Distension of the abdomen; anxiety, with a feeling of flying heat internally, and stupefaction of the head; somnolence; antiperistaltic motion of the intestines; constant vomiting and belching; retention of stool and urine; complete inactivity of the lower bowels.

Rhus Tox :—Great restlessness; changing position, notwithstanding the pain it causes; tongue red at the tip; pressive cutting pain in the abdomen; typhoid symptoms; febris lente; metritis.

Sulphur :—After Aconite or Bryonia, or when the disease takes a protracted course.

Veratrum :—Vomiting and diarrhoea; coldness of the skin; sunken features; pulse small and weak; thirst great; restlessness and anxiety.

——

CHAPTER XXXVII

ACUTE PELVIC CELLULITIS

ACUTE PELVIC CELLBULITIS Means an acute inflammation of the pelvic cellular tissues.

Aetiology

1. Infected cervix, extending the infection to the cellular tissues through posterior fornix.
2. Trauma or injury.
3. Post-childbirth or abortion; i.e., Septic condition occuring after delivery.
4. Secondary to pelvic penitonitis or salpingitis.
5. Organisms responsible are only the pyogenic bacteria.

Signs And Symptoms

1. Cellulitis is milder than Peritonitis; so, there is insidious rise of temperature, as compared to Peritonitis.
2. Dull pain in the lower abdomen and back.
3. Vomiting is absent.
4. Temperature and toxaemia are less marked.
5. Tenderness and rigidity of the abdomen also less marked or may be absent, because, here, the deeper tissues are involved.
6. On P.V. examination :
   Hard tender swelling in one or both the lateral fornices or rarely if pus forms, fluctuation may be found.
7. On rectal examination :
   A horse-shoe shaped swelling is felt around the rectum: lerving aside the posterior side, it is present on all the three sides, and that is a characteristic sign of cellulitis.

Prognosis

Prognosis is always good; of course, it may have certain complications

Courses And Complications

The effusion gets absorbed during the treatment.

When abscess forms, it may point out or even burst into any area—into the rectum, vagina, inguinal region or hip or elsewhere; it has to be drained out in any case. After that, it may be dissolved with the homoeopathic drugs.

Treatment

1. Bed rest.
2. Light and nutritious diet.
3. Modern antibiotic treatment.
4. Alkaline mixtures.
5. Sedatives for allaying the pains.
6. Then, the homoeopathic remedies.
   Aco., Ars., Bell., Bry., Hepar S.. Merc. Sol., Sulphur, or any other remedy depending upon the symptoms.

THERAPEUTIC HINTS

Aconite :—Usual febrile symptoms with restlessness, mental agony and fear of death; anxious expression of face; burning, cutting, darting pains in the bowels, worse slightest pressure, motion and lying on right side; abdomen hot to touch; after violent emotions which have checked the flow of lochia, after checked sweat, exposure to dry cold wind or drinking cold water when heated.

Arsemic :—Abdomen enormously distended, feels as if it would burst; unquenchable thirst; lancinating and burning pains, wishes to to be kept warm by wraps and hot applications; great mental distress, fears death sudden sinking of strength; cold clammy sweat; rapid emaciation; worse after midnight.

Belladonna :—Abdomen distended, hot and exquisitely tender to touch or to the least jar of bed; pains in sudden attacks, coming and going suddenly or less frequently, gradually increase and gradually decrease; high temperature, on raising sheets a hot steam rises; head hot and dry or hot and sweating; feet cold; urine scanty and golden-yellow; delirium to drowsiness and stuper; face pale, hot, cold cheeks and hot forehead, sweat only on face; red face with starting, anxious look, expressive of deep-seated distress; drowsiness and stupor, but easily, aroused. In complication with metritis, lochia checked or hot in offensively smeliing clots, back feels as if broken. In complication with enteritis or typhlitis, clutching as from nails around the navel, bloody, slimy diarrhoea.

Bryonia :—Complication with diaphragmitis; stitching, pressing, lancinating pains in the bowels with each breath, worse from slightest motion; tongue white down centre and dry; can only breathe in short, quick inspirations, hence features express great anguish; great thirst; bowels constipated, urine scanty, dark-red and clear.

Hepar-Suplh. :—Attended with uterine ulcers, having bloody suppuration, smelling like old cheese; edge of ulcer sensitive; often a pulsating sensation in ulcers; much itching or little pimples around the ulcer; discharge of blood between the periods; leucorrhoea, with smarting of vulva. Patient is highly sensitive to cold, cold air; every draft of cold air brings on the complaints. Pain, tenderness in the lower abdomen, with feeling of pulsation, threatening pus-formation.

Merc. Sol. :—After Belladonna, when suppuration commences, with tympanitic abdomen, serous or purulent effusion, sweat, rigors. On os uteri bleeding excrescenes, or deep ulcers with ragged edges; plolapsus uteri, deep sore pain in the pelvis; dragging in the loins; abdomen feels weak, as if it had to be help up; griping and bruised pain in small of back; painful pressure in the thighs; itching of genitals, worse from contact of urine; leucorrhoea smarting, corroding, causing itching, or purulent, containing lumps, worse at night. Great perspiration, but that does not relieve the suffering. All complaints worse at night, heat of bed. History of syphilis or gonorrhoea is often traced.

Rhus Tox :—Great restlessness, changing position, though it increases the pain; weakness; tongue red, dry; red at the tip; tympany; low muttering dellirium; her dreams are full of laborious efforts; pressing, cutting pain in abdomen; typhoid state, metritis with septicaemia; in complication with enteritis, bloody stools, with tearing down the thighs; pulse accelerated, irregular or intermittent.

Sulphur :—Leading to peritonitis even, especially after puerperium, at its commencement right off asthenic; limbs go to sleep, great lassitude and weariness. Prolapsus from reaching high up, worse from standing, with pain in right hypogastrium; bearing down in the pelvis towards genitals; weak feeling in hypogastrium and genitals; sore feeling in vagina during embrace; itching of vulva with pimples all round and burning in vagina; uterine pains running from groins to back; sterility with too early and profuse menses; corroding yellow leucorrhoea, preceded by pain in the abdomen.

Consult the remedies discussed under CHRONIC-PELVIC-CELLULITIS also.

——

CHAPTER XXXVIII

CHRONIC PELVIC CELLULITIS

CHRONIC PELVIC CELLULITIS is the chronic inflammation and a low grade infection of the pelvic cellular tissues. Cellular tissues are the deep structures, which have no nerve supply, of course.

Aetiology :

1. As a sequela of the acute inflammation of cellular tissues of the pelvis.
2. And, all other causes mentioned under the aetiology of Acute pelvic cellulitis.

In this condition, certain amount of fibrosis is present with adhesions occuring as a result of the acute inflammation. Due to these adhesions the uterus becomes immobile.

Signs and Symptoms :

1. History of some acute inflammation in the past is often traceable; such as, salpingitis, peritonitis, cervicitis, etc.
2. Pain in the ingiunal and iliac regions on pressure.
3. Dysmenorrhoea, i.e., painful menstruation due to congestion of the uterus.
4. Lecorrhoea, is generally present when any of the generative organs is infected and inflamed.
5. Dyspareunia, i.e., painful coition may also be there due to the inflammation of surrounding tissues.
6. On P.V. examination :
   (i) Uterus is immoble (probably due to adhesions).
   (ii) Solid masses are felt in the lateral fornices.
   (iii) Movement of the cervix causes pain when it is moved on the affected side.

(iv) Cervical erosion may be present, since it is the primary focus.

Treatment

As far as the adhesions are concerned, they can be and are removed surgically.

For other symptoms, suitable homoeopathic remedies are given on thé basis of totality of characteristic symptos and the constitution of the individual patient.

Calc. Carb., Calc. Fluor, Conium, Graph., Lach., Apis, Brom., Ustilago, Puls., Murex, Platina, Podo., Iod., Phos., Merc. Sol., Sulph. and Silicea.

THERAPEUTIC HINTS

Calcarea Carb. :—Abdomen much distended and hard; frequent severe cramps in the bowels with coldness of thighs, worse by cold water, so that the patient wants the cold wet compresses constantly renewed; urine dark, without sediment constipation. Prolapse with sensation of pressure on the uterus, bearing-down pains, worse when standing; stinging in os, burning in cervical canal, constant aching in the vagina; polypi; backache, heaviness of limbs and great fatigue from walking; desire for sweets or boiled eggs. Patient is fat, fair and flabby, with much sweat.

Calcarea Flour. :—Great depression, groundless fears of financial ruins. Indicision. Displacements of uterus with dragging pain in the region of the uterus and thighs, bearing-down of the uterus. Varicose veins of the vulva. Swelling felt very hard on examination. Menses are profuse and ulcer formation with hardened edges.

Conium :—With induration and enlargement of ovaries, with lancinating pains; stinging in neck of uterus; induration and prolapsus at the same time; frequent nausea, vomiting; acrid and burning leucorrhoea, preceded by pinching pains in the abdomen; sensation of debility in the morning when in bed; sudden loss of strength while walking; chronic pressive inflammation of ovaries; ovarian depression with scanty menses and sterility; pressive and cutting pains in uterus when urinating; weight and lancinating pains in ovaries and uterus extending through lower part of the abdomen, hips and back; burning, stinging, darting pains in neck of the womb, with scirrhous indurations.

Graphtes :—Cancer of the womb, with warmth and painfulness of vagina, engorgement of lymphantic vessels and mucous follicles, hardness of neck of womb, which is swollen and covered with fungus excrescences ; heaviness of abdomen, with exacerbation of pains and fainting while standing ; stitches through thighs and hypogastrium, like electric shocks ; retarded and painful menses, with discharge of back, coagulated and foetid blood, constipation, earthy complexion, sadness and restlessness. Tumour, size of an orange, in right and left iliac fossa, hard, round, slightly moveable, not painful to pressure, only producing inconvenience from weight ; os uteri standing backward, can only be reached with difficulty ; pain in uterus when reaching high with arms ; bearing-down pains in uterus to back, with weakness and sickness ; vagina cold ; cicatrical tissue easily craces and bleeds.

Lachesis :—Inflameq caecum, abdomen hot, and even if unconscious she will resist the slightest touch to abdomen ; painful stiffness from loins down to thighs ; scanty, turbid urine, with reddish sediment ; strangury; constipation or tormenting urging in rectum ; parts most distant from heart cool ; pulse rapid, feeble, intermittent ; tonguc trembless and catches behind the lower teeth : lies on back with knees drawn up ; arouses from sleep smothering.

Apis :—Distressing aching soreness of abdomen which will toletrate no pressure, or sudden knife-like stabs through abdomen ; urine scanty, dark, albuminous ; absence of thirst or drinks little and often ; oedematous puffing of face; sleepy, but cannot sleep from nervousness and fidgetiness.

Bromium :—Continual dull pain in left ovary ; no thrill in coition; swelling and hardness of left ovary ; uterus descends about two inches ; loud emission of flatus from vagina ; membranous dysmenorrhoca ; vertigo with fear of falling and losing their senses.

Ustilago :—Constant aching, referred to mouth of womb; displaced uterus with menorrhagia ; cervix tunefied, bleeds when touched, for days oozing of dark blood, with small coagula; bearing down as if everything would come through ; menses profuse, frequent containing coagula ; goneness in epigastrium ; sub-involution; fibroid tumours.

Pulsatilla :—Prolapsus uteri, worse on lying down and from heat, better in fresh air with pressure in abdomen and small of back as from a stone ; limbs tend to go to sleep ; ineffectual urging to stool ; suppressed menses, pains in back and chilliness; cramp constiriction in vagina ; peevishness, with weeping ; dimness of vision ; pressure on bladder, frequent and copious micturition, without and strangury.

Murex :—Prolapsus with uterine pains extending upward from right side of uterus, crossing the body to the left mamma; pain in uterus as if cut by a sharp instrument; uterus feels dry, as if constricted ; myalgic pain in uterus, coming on when in bed, better by sitting or walking. until tired out, when she must lie down from temporary relief, as the cutting pains come on again, going through her up diagonally, compelling her to get up again and walk, feeling as if something were pressing on a sore spot in the pelvis ; venereal desire so violent as to fatigue reason, renewed by slightest touch ; green or bloody leucorrhoea ; profuse menses ; gone sensation in the stomach worse about 11 in forenoon, better by eating and lying down ; frequent urination at night, urine pale, wakes with a start and violent desire to urinate; muscular debility and mental depression.

Platina :—Induration of uterus ; ulceration, with coexisting ovarian irritation ; nymphomania ; tingling or titillation from genitals up into abdomen ; metrorrhagia, with great excitability of sexual system ; pruritus vulvae, with anxiety and palpitation of heart ; prolapsus uteri, with continual pressure in genital organs ; numbness and coldness of body ; melancholy ; great sensitiveness of genitals, it hurts her to sit down ; neuralgia uteri.

Podophyllum :—Prolapsus uteri at vagina after straining or overlifting, after parturition, with pain in sacrum ; prolapsus ani with torpid liver and constipation; much bearing down in hypogastric and sacral region, increased by motion and relieved by lying down ; numb, aching pains in ovaries, particularly on left side ; sensation as if genitals would protrude during stool, even during diarrhoea, with leucorrhoea of thick, transparent mucus; fulness of superficial veins; menorrhagia from straining.

Iodium :—Induration and swelling of uterus and ovaries; dropsical affection of ovaries, with pressing down towards genitals; cancerous degeneration of neck of uterus; acrid leucorrhoea, corroding the limbs, worse at the time of menses; uterine haemorrhage, renewed at every stool; numb feeling in thighs and legs; emaciation, hectic fever, canine hunger or no appetite; constipation or looseness of bowels.

Phosphorus :—In complication with peritonitis having tymparites, abdomen excessively sensitive to touch; burning and pressure in abdomen; sharp, cutting pains in abdomen Endometritis; prolapsus with weak, sinking feeling in abdomen; uterine pains running upward; stitches from vagina into pelvis, sterility from excessive volup-tuousness, or with profuse and too late menses; corroding leucorrhoea instead of menses, causing blisters; cancer of uterus, with frequent and profuse flooding, pouring out freely and then ceasing for a short time; emaciation and nervous debility; hyperaesthesia, frequent fainting.

Silicea :—Nymphomania, with spinal affections, nausea after an embrace; very little sexual desire; prolapsus uteri from myelitis; serous cysts in vagina; itching of genitals; pressing-down feeling in vagina, parts tender to touch; irregular menses, flow strong-smelling, acrid; bloody discharge between the periods; profuse, acrid, corroding leucorrhoea; amenorrhoea with suppressed foot-sweat or metrorrhagia; hysteria; great debility.

Remedies discussed under ACUTE-PELVIC-CELLULITIS should also be studied.

——

CHAPTER XXXIX
PELVIC ABSCESS

PELVIC ABSCESS is an abscess of the cellular tissues of the pelvis and in the pouch of Doughlas.

Aetiology :

It may follow acute salpingitis, acute pelvic pertitonitis and cellulitis, rupture of pyosalpinx or appendical abscess, infection of the cervix or any other pyogenic bacterial infection.

Signs and Symptoms

It remains confined to the pelvis by adhesions which separate it from the peritoneum.

1. Usually, there is high temperature, coming on in the night.
2. Pulse rate is raised.
3. Perspiration.
4. Sometimes, there is a feeling of pain in the pelvic region.
5. Feeling of fullness or discomfort in the pelvis.
6. Pain and tenderness in the lower abdomen, and as a result, the patient resists the physical examination, especially the P.V. examination.
7. Flatulent swelling felt in the pouch of Doughlas, which may be pressing on the vagina and possibly trying to point in that direction.

Treatment :

1. When the abscess forms, it has to be drained out in order to effect an early healing.
2. After that, suitable homoeopathic remedies should be given on the basis of the totality of peculiar symptoms of the patient.

Bell., Bry., Heper S., Merc. Sol., Sulph., Puls., Graph., Calc Carb., Calc Phos., etc.

THEREPEUTIC HINTS

Belladonna :—It is the remedy most often indicated for the initiatory symptoms of abscess. The parts swell rapidly, become bright red, there is intense throbbing which is painful pus develops speedily, the swelling increases and the redness radiates. It corresponds more closely to the active, sthenic variety of abscess before pus is matured. The abdomen is swollen, which is tense like a drum, very sensitive to touch, so sensitive that the patient wants the bed-clothes removed. The least jar greatly aggravates. There is pungent heat of the body, it seems to steam out on raising the bed-clothes ; the abdomen especially the lower portion is intensely hot. There is much cerebral irritation, perhaps delirium and the discharge is scanty or suppressed. The slightest noise, loud talking and light aggravate. The patient is uneasy ; must constantly change her position, but is made worse thereby. There is a sensation as if the bowels were grasped or clawed and a violent pressure towards the genital organs; the latter symptom is almost a deciding one. There is also a continued distressful retching, and vomiting even of bile.

Bryonia :—It is indicated when the fever is violent with a burning heat all over ; the patient is in an impatient irascible mood and the excitability of the nervous system is marked. There is violent thirst. The patient drinking much and probably vomiting it soon afterwards. The patient is alternately chilly and hot, with sharp stitching pains in the abdomen, worse from pressure and motion. The abdomen is also swollen, hot and sensitive ; there is constipation and the patient has a yellowish gray complexion.

Calcarea Carb. :—Pressing on the uterus ; aching of the vagina ; stinging in the os uteri ; the menses appear too soon and are too profuse ; milk-like leucorrhoea ; inclination to perspire easily about the head, great liability to strain a part by lifting; easily tired by bodily exertions ; in walking upstairs, she feels dizzy and entirely exhausted; even talking makes her weak ; great inclination to sign ; she cannot get her breath long enough ; great susceptibility to catch cold ; the feet feel most of the time damp and cold, or else the soles of the feel are burning hot ; great desire for hard boiled eggs or sweets; big-belliedness; scrofulous diathesis.

Calcarea Phos :—Prolapses, worse during defaecation and micturition, with sense of weakness and distress ; aching in womb ; cutting pain through sacrum ; cervix and os swollen, red and painful, with feeling of shot-like bundles to digital touch; burning in vagina and burning like fire upward into chest ; flushes of heat, anxiety, faintness; joints ache at every change of the weather; easy perspiration ; polypi.

Graphites :—Perfectly white discharge, very profuse, especially in the morning on rising from bed, also in gushes by day or night ; scanty menses, irritable skin ; weakness in back and small of back when walking or sitting. Caul-flower excrescence ; burning stitching pains, like electric shocks, through the womb, extending into the thighs; great heaviness in the abdomen when standing, with incraesed pains and faintness; menses only every six weeks ; with a discharge of black, clotted, offensive blood, and an increase of all the sufferings ; constipation; earthy colour of the face ; frequent chilliness; sad, despondings. The patient is obese, with tendency to skin affections.

Hepar Sulph :—It is the great homoeopathic remedy for suppurations where the pus is not decomposed. It suits epecially to the lymphatic, phlegmatic individuals. Excessive sensitiveness of the part is a leading indication; chilly sensations, throbbing in the parts, or sharp, sticking pains which are worse at night and from cold.

Lachesis :—Here, the pus is thin, dark, ichorous and offensive. It is the remedy for abscess where poisonous matter has been introduced into the system, cousing the trouble. The fever is worse at night. The slightest touch to the surface of the abdomen, particularly the lower portion of it, is unbearable. There is tenderness present at one spot. The gangrenous tendency is marked under this remedy.

Mercurius Sol. :—It comes in after Belladonna, when pus has formed ; the pus is greenish in tint, and quite thin and fluid. There is intense shining redness with throbbing and stinging pains. The abdomen is tympanitic, showing the evidence of seropurulent matter present, and the patient has rigors and sweats. There is night aggravation, the desire for cold water, rumbling in abdomen and the diarrhoeic stools. Frequent exacerbating fever with creeping chills and copious perspiration, with no relief.

Pulsatilla :—Prolapsus uteri, worse on lying down and from heat, better in fresh air, with pressure in abdomen and small of back as from a stone ; limbs tend to go to sleep ; ineffectual urging to stool ; suppressed menses, pains in back and chilliness; cramp constriction in vagina ; peevishness with weeping; dimness of vision; pressure on bladder, frequent and copious micturition, without any strangury. The discharge of pus is thick, bland and yellowish-green. Thirstless. She wants her head high ; feels uncomfortable with only one pillow. We can very often, trace the history of gonorrhoea in such cases.

Silicea :—It is the remedy where the suppuration continues and the wound refuses to heal; the pus is apt to be thin, watery, and the process is a sluggish and indolent one. It is usually given after an abscess has been lanced or opened by means of a poultice. The patient feels much better with warmth. There is much cellular infiltration round the abscess. The discharge of pus is considerably foetid.

Sulphur :—It is especially useful in chronic cases where the discharge is profuse and accompanied with emaciation and hectic fever. The pus is acrid and excoriating. It is to be thought of when the rightly selected remedy fails to give the desired result. In association with prolapsus of the uterus from reaching high, worse from standing, with pain in the hypogastrium on the right side ; bearing down in pelvis towards the genitals ; weak feeling in hypogastrium and genitals ; sore feeling in vagina during embrace ; itching of vulva, with pimples all round and burning in vagina ; uterine pains running from groins to back ; sterility with too early and profuse menses; corroding yellow leucorrhoea, preceded by pain in the abdomen.

——

CHAPTER XXXX

DISEASES OF THE BREASTS

MASTITIS

1. Mastitis of infancy.
2. Mastitis of puberty.
3. Mastitis due to local irritation in the nipple and areola.
4. Mastitis of lactation.
5. Suppurative Mastitis.
6. Chronic mastitis.

1. **Mastitis of Infancy :**—It is seen on the 3rd or 4th day of life which occurs on account of hormonal effect of the mother. The symptom is the oozing of milk-like-fluid on pressing the nipple of the child alongwith a little swelling underneath. The condition becomes mormal in about 3-4 weeks time or the milk is squeezed out.

Mastitis of Puberty :—It is present at the time of puberty, of course in both sexes. It occurs on accout of hormonal imbalance taking place at that time. There is tenderness and slight pain in the breast. It is the usual course and is alright in due course of time.

3, **Mastitis due to Local Irritation in the Nipple and Areola :**—It occurs as a result of wearing of tight brassiers showing its presence by pain and tenderness.

4. **Mastitis of lactation :**—It is also known as acute mastitis or spilt-milk mastitis. It occurs due to inadequate feeding because the sucking power of the child is inefficient; the epithelial cells block the milk ducts. If the obstruction is not removed, the milk is collected in the alveoli, they expand and may burst causing the milk to spread into the surrounding breast tissue ; then there is severe pain, redness, signs of inflammation and fever. At this stage there is no pus. The affection is usually seen after the first delivery.

Treatment

Treatment is massage, adequate evacuation of milk manually or by the breast pump and the indicated remedies.

5. **Suppurative Mastilis** :—It may occur due to improperly treated mastitis or cracked nipples through which infection gets in and causes the pus to form. The condition is diagnosed by T.L.C. and D.L C. and fluctuation. T.L.C. may increase with a relative increase in the Polymorphs.

Treatment lies in drawing out of the pus through Surgical means and then the indicated anti-suppurative medicines.

6. **Chronic Mastitis** :—In this condition there is no pus formation but there is evidence of inflammation as detected by the histological examination of the breast tissue. It occurs in the middle aged women from 35-45 years, in unmarried or childless women.

Remedies :

Bell.; Bry., Phytolacca, Hepar Sulph., Merc., Puls., Sulphur, Fluoric Acid, Cham., Phos., etc.

THERAPEUTIC HINTS

Apis :—Burning, stinging pain in the breasts; considerable swelling and hardness; erysipelatous inflammation.

Arnica :—Soreness of the nipples; bruises of the breasts,

Belladonna :—During nursing and weaning, great hardness and swelling; bright redness in streaks along the milk-ducts; throbbing, stitching pain; headace; fever; worse in the afternoon; bowels constipated, and urine scanty.

Bryonia ;—Mastitis sets in mostly with a chill, followed by fever; great stitching pain in the breast, worse from slightest motion; tense swelling; little or no redness, bursting pain in the head when rising, with dizziness; great thirst; thick coated tongue; constipation; faeces as if burnt; pain in all the limbs when moving.

Graphites :—Inflamed, cracked nipples; tettery eruptions on the scalp, hands and between the fingers, indurated Meibomian glands; old cicatrices from former inflammations.

Hamamelis :—Bleeding nipples, with great soreness.

Hepar Sulph :—Pain in the upper arms and thighs, as if in the bones, great hastiness in drinking and speaking; also in persons who have taken a great deal of mercury; when suppuration commences with frequent crawls, or when, after the breaking or opening of the abscesses the discharge is scanty and there still remains great hardness of the inflamed parts.

Lachesis :—When the inflamed breast has a purplish appearance.

Mercurius :—Especially when after Belladonna, notwithstand suppuration sets in; chilliness and profuse sweat, which does not relieve; great nervous weakness and trembling; also in cases where suppuration takes place in different parts of the breast.

Nux vomica :—Nipples painful during suckling, with little or no soreness or rawness.

Phosphorus :—Phlegmonous inflammation; breast swollen; red in spots or streaks; hard knots in different places, with fistulous opening, discharging a watery, discoloured, offensive ichor; dry, hacking cough, with hectic fever and colliquative sweats; slender built women, with a white and tender skin; weakened by disease or loss of fluids.

Phytolacca :—Sore and fissured nipples, with intense suffering when putting the child to the breast; the pain seems to start from the nipple and irradiate all over the body going to the backbone, and streaking up and down, with excessive flow of milk, causing great exhaustion; a few days after confinement sudden chill, followed by some fever and a painful engorgement, and swelling of the mammae; the drawing of milk is impossible. In ordinary caked breasts it is called specific. Badly-treated "gathered breast" with large, fistulous, gaping and angry ulcers filled with unhealthy granulations and discharging a watery, ichorous pus; the gland is full of hard, painful nodosities.

Rhus tox. :—Soreness and swelling of the breast from taking cold, especially getting wet; pain in all the limbs; worse when at rest; great restlessness; the lochial discharge turns red again.

Silicea :—Chronic cases ; when Phosphorus is not sufficient to heal the fistulous opening with callous edges, or to disperse the hard lumps in the breast ; pale, earthy colour in the fa loss of smell; hectic fever.

Croton Tig. :—Pains shoot from the nipples to the shoulders.

Phellandrium :—Stitching pain in nipples and pain along the milk ducts.

Pulsatilla :—An excellent remedy for scanty or abscence of milk ; the patient is gloomy or tearful. It is useful where mechanical irritation excites the flow of milk in young girls.

Urtica Urens :—Non-appearance of milk, with no special symptoms.

Sulphur :—Sore and cracked nipples, with bleeding when nursing, the areolae are covered with yellowish scale from underneath of which oozes an acrid fluid, with itching and burning in the night ; hard lumps in the breast ; ulcerating sore, with spongy excrescences and great itching ; sleepless nights.

— —

TUMOURS

TUMOUR is an abnormal new growth of tissues which is functionless and harmful to the body. It is also called **Neoplasm**.

It is differentiated from **hypertrophy**, which means a uniform development of tissue, with corresponding increase of function.

It is also differentiated from **inflmmation** or **inflmmatory** Swelling which is due to congestion of the blood and inflammatory process followed by absorption and formation of connective tissues. It has redness; heat, pain and loss of function.

Oedema pits on pressure and may occur over a large part of the body; whereas, tumour is localised and does not pit on pressure.

A **cyst** being filled with fluid, yields to pressure ; but, a tumour is solid and will not yield to pressure.

Hyperplasia is the result of injury and inflammation and is due to reparatory process of the tissues, and the tumour is an independent growth and is not under the law of growth.

The tumours resemble a parasitic condition to the host, because they survive and develop on the blood of the person. They have no function, but they can produce harm by pressure upon the adjoining tissues and organs.

Aetiology

1. Age :—Age has a great influence in the development of tumours. The malignant tumour, like carinoma, is an affection of the old age, generally 40 years and above, whereas sarcoma generally occurs in the earlier periods of life.

2. Sex :—Both sexes are liable to the growth of tumor but in females, there are certain organs which are more commonly affected ; e. g., uterus, cervix and mammary glands.

3. **Occupation** :– There are some occupations which lead to the tumour formation, e. g., chimney-sweepers are more prone to the occurance of lung cancer.

4. **Habits** :— Certain habits, like continuous smoking, lead to the formation of lung cancer.

5. **Heredity** :–In certain families, cancer occurs in a number of relatives belonging to that family.

6. **Constant irritation after injuries** :—It has been observed that tumours grow commonly after some injury or irritation; e.g., adenoma of the breast, sarcoma developnig after injuries and carcinoma of lips from irritation of clay pipes of smokers.

It has also been observed that irritation due to heat of charcoal carried by Kashmiris near their abdomen and thighs produces cancer at the site of chronic burns.

There are some chemicals which irritate the tissues to produce cancer; e. g.; coal tar, shale oil, soot, etc.

Prolonged exposure to X-ray and radium also causes cancer.

Dietetic deficiencies may also lead to the formation of cancer; e.g., cancer of the liver, though a rare disease in most of the countries, is very common in Java and the Bantus of South Africa. This may be due to the deficiency of some element in diet.

Cancer of cervix in women and of lungs in men is much more common amongst the poor cleasses.

Cancer of larynx is, more often, found in singers, actors and clergymen.

7. **Endogenous Factors** :— There are some sex hormones which produce disordered metabolism and act as cancer producing substances. Oestrin acts on the mammary epithelium which is normally under the influence of ovarian stimulation. It has been observed that if oestrin is injected from birth onwards into a strain of mice which have a natural tendency to develop mammary cancer, the incidence of that tumour is greatly increased. It is important to note that in non-cancerous

strain, the hormone is powerless to produce cancer. Removal of the ovaries in mice of a high cancer strain will prevent the occurance of spontaneous mammary cancer.

These factors suggest the possibility that the hormones may be a conditioning factor to the production of cancer. It is probable that the male sex hormone plays some part in the production of cancer of the prostate.

Morphology of Tumours

1. **Composition** :—The tumour is composed of specific cells or tissues of the body. The tumour cells resemble closely the normal cells histologically.

2. **Size** :—The size of tumour varies from a pin-head to an enormous size. It depends upon the type of tumour and the growth of tumour.

3. **Shape** :—The general shape of the tumour is spherical (oval); but, it may be of any other shape.

4. **Consistency** :—It depends upon the cells involved; e.g., a lipoma, which is due to the growth of fatty-tissues, is of soft consistency, whereas a bone tumour will be very hard on account of its origin from thé bone.

5. **Number** :—Tumour may be single or they may be multiple at the same time.

6. **Vascularity** :—The tumours are richly supplied with blood vassels and lymphatics; but there are no nerves inside the tumour.

7. **Growth** :—The tumour cells have unceasing growth and multiplication. Their growth is autonomous, i. e., it is not affected by external influences. It depends opon the cellular activity independently. They can grow from any kind of tissue of the body.

8. **Disposition** :—The tumours are either benign or malignant according to their tendency to malignancy.

Classification

The tumours may be classified into three varieties :—

1. **Benign** :—They are generally tissue tumours ; they are simple and so are not so harmful.

2. Malignant :—They are the cell tumours; they generally grow rapidly, are very harmful and may cause death of the person. They are further classified into :

(a) Carcinoma, and

(b) Sarcoma.

3. Mixed tumours :—They show a variety of tissues and cells in the tumour, e. g., teratoma.

BENIGN TUMOURS

The following varieties of Benign tumours are commonly found.

Osteoma., Chondroma, Myoma, Fibroma, Glioma, Haemangioma, Lymphangioma, Adenoma, Papiloma, and Lipoma.

Name of Tumour	Name of tissue	Location
1. Osteoma	Bone	Skull, face and nasal cavities.
2. Chondroma	Cartilage.	Pelvic bone certilage, larynx and bronchi.
3. Myoma.	Muscle fibres.	Uterus, urinary bladder and stomach.
4. Fibroma, Neurofibroma & Myxofibroma.	Fibrous-strands of collagen. fibres.	Occurs in the form of subcutaneous molluscum fibrosum, known as Rickling--hausen's disease : Left auricle of heart.
5. Glioma	Brain cells.	Intracranial tumours are formed of glioma.
6. Haemangioma.	Blood vessels.	Capillaries and blood vessels of face, lips, tongue, liver and brain.
7. Lymphangioma.	Lymphatic vessels.	Tongue, neck and axilla.

Name of Tumour	Name of tissue	Location
8. Adenoma	Glandular tissues	Thyroid, supra--renal glands, pancreas, kidneys.
9. Papiloma	Mucous membrane	Nose, larynx, vulva, uterus and cervix.
10. Lipoma	Fatty tissues	Subcutaneous tissues of skin, back and shoulders and sometimes the mesentery.

MALIGNANT TUMOURS

CARCINOMA

A carcinoma is a malignant epithelial tumour which tends to invade the lymph spaces of the surrounding connective tissues. It is the commonest of all the malignant tumours. The cells show the characteristic epithelial arrangement. The fibrous stroma acts as a supporting frame work for the epithetical cells.

Carcinoma originates primarily from any tissue containing the epithelium. As a matter of fact, no tissue is exempt from the secondary growth of carcinoma. The primary growth occurs in the skin, breast, uterus, alimentary canal, respiratory tract, liver, pancreas and all other organs where epithelium is present.

Morphology

The morphology of carcinoma is variable. Carcinomas vary in size, shape and general appearance. Generally, three main forms are recognized.

Nodular,

Ulcerative, and

Fungating forms.

Carinoma may develop necrosis, degeneration and fibrosis causing great distortion to the appearance of the tumour.

In the nodular form, the tumour may be round or irregular in shape and hard in consistency.

The ulcerative form is most common when the tumour is superficial, as in case of skin, breast, stomach, etc.

The fungating form is characterized by masses of foul small, redness, easy bleeding and suppurating tissue.

The colour of these tumours is generally grey or white.

Histology

The cancer cells are derived from the epithelial cells of the affected organ. The cell-arrangement depends upon the type of carcinoma.

Spread of Carcinoma

1. By invasion of the tissue spaces.
2. By lymphatic permeation : the cancer cells invade the lymphatics and grow along them.
3. By lymphatic embolism : the tumour cells are carried to the lymph nodes, and sometimes, to more distant nodes.
4. By blood stream : the tumour cells may be carried to distant organs by the blood stream.

In cancer of gastro-intestinal canal and pancreas, the tumour emboli are carried by the portal vein to the liver to form metastasis. The bones are frequently the site of metastasis in carcinoma of the prostate, breasts, lungs, kidneys and thyroid.

Classification of Carcinoma

1. Squamous-Cell Carcinoma :—It is also called epithelioma and occurs on the skin, mucous membrane of the mouth, lips, tongue, face, eyelids, nose, pharynx, larynx, gall-bladder, urinary bladder, penis, anus, labia, vagina, cervix and uterus.

The tumour consists of squamous epithelium arranged in masses invading the deeper layers with disorganisation of the basement membrane. The newly formed cells are observed. The oldest cells occupy the central position and undergo a change known as **keratosis** or **hornygrowth**. The peripheral cells are present in large masses joined together by means of a large number of protoplasmic outgrowths or prickles. These cells are loaded with black-staining droplets of eleidin similar to keratin. The keratinisation and prickle cells are characteristic of squasmous cell carcinoma. Round cell infiltration is present, in considerable degree, in the stroma. The presence of a large number of plasma cells is common.

2 **Adeno Carcinoma :**—It is also known as glandular-cell-carcinoma. It develops from the glandular cells of parotid glands, thyroid gland, pancreas and mammary glands ; but, it is, most commonly, found in the breasts. The cells are usually spheroidal in shape but often become polygonal due to mutal pressure. The cells possess an abundant cytoplasm with a deeply stained nucleus. They are grouped in columns or in solid alveoli according to the organ affected. The tumour is not of rapid growth. The dense stroma make the tumour very hard and is called scirrhus. But, when the stroma is scanty and delicate the tumour is soft and is called encephaloid or medullary. The encephaloid variety appears softer and shows more rapid growth than the scirrhus variety. Both varieties generally occur in the breasts, ovaries and stomach.

3. **Basal Cell Carcinoma :**—The lesion occurs in the basal layer of epidermis especially on the face, eyes and lips. It causes ulceration and infiltrates in the surrounding tissues, but does not give out metastasis.

It is relatively benign, of remarkably slow growth and does not involve regional lympth glands. Exposure to bright sunlight appears to be an exciting factor.

It consists of solid masses of darkly stained cells which extend down into the dermis. The columns extend down to a uniform level and their ends have a expanded club shaped appearance. Melanin pigment may be abundant. The line of demarcation between the epithelium and the stroma is sharply defined indicating a benign type of growth.

The ulcer, in this variety, is known as 'Rodent Ulcer;

4. **Mucinoid Carcinoma :**—It develops from the secreting cells in the mucous membrane of the stomach, intestines, gall bladder, bile ducts, pancreas and body of the uterus.

The tumour resembles the glandular tissue with definite alveolar arrangement although irregular. The glandular arrangement is often modified in the metastatic growths, but the presence of the columnar cells can be made out on careful examination in such secondary growths. It spreads both by the lymphatics and blood stream. The change from the normal mucous membrane of the bowel to irregular glands of the tumour, is very sudden.

5. Transitional Cell Carcinoma :— It develops from the urinary tract and naso–pharynx.

SARCOMA

Sarcoma is another variety of malignant tumours. These are generally the tissue tumours originating from the connective tissues of the body. They spread through the blood stream, lymphatic vessels and local infiltration The age of occurance is below 40 years; i. e., the occurance of sarcoma is an affection of young people below 40 years. This type of tumours is of rare variety.

Classification

They are of the same type as the benign tumours; when the tumour becomes malignant, it is known as sarcoma.

Name of Tumour	Neme of Tissue	Location
1. Osteosarcoma.	Bone.	Skull bone, face and nasal cavities.
2. Chondrosarcoma.	Cartilage	Pelvic bone cartilage, larynx and bronchi.
3. Myosacroma	Muscle fibres.	Uterus, urinary bladder and stomach.
4. Fibrosarcoma	Fibrous tissues.	Subcutaneous molluscum fibrosum.
5. Gliosarcoma	Brain tissue.	Cranium.
6. Haemangiosarcoma	Blood vessels.	Capillaries and blood vessels of face, lips, tongue and liver.

Name of Tumour	Name of Tissue	Location
7. Lymphangiosarcoma	Lymphatic vessels.	Tongue, neck and axilla.
8. Adenosarcoma	Glandular tissues	Thyroid, supra-renals, pancreas, kidneys.
9 Papilosarcoma	Mucous membrane.	Nose, larynx, vulva, uterus, and cervix.
10. Liposarcoma.	Fatty tissues.	Subcutaneous tissues of skin, back and shoulders and sometimes of the mesentery.

MIXED TUMOURS

These tumours show a variety of tissues and cells in them, e. g., Teratoma.

Teratoma

A teratoma is a tumour derived from all the three blasto'-dermic germinal layers. A malignant growth may develop in a teratoma and may be carcinomatous or sarcomatous in type They occur commonly in the form of dermoid cysts, mixed parotid tumours, congenital sacro-coccygeal growth and teratoma of the testes.

These tumours often become cystic and contain the following elements :

1. Epiblastic element, e. g., hair follicles. sweat glands, sebaceous glands, teeth nerve firbres, mucous membrane and skin.
2. Mesoblastic element ; e. g., areolar tissue, muscles, cartilage and bone, etc.
3. Hypoblastic element; e. g., endothelium.

Every grade of complexity may be met within a teratoma. It is not a tumour in the strict sense of the word, but, rather an attempted formation of a new individual within the tissues of the patient. In the early stage of development and segmenting ovum, a mutation occurs resulting in the formation of this kind of tumour.

Benign Tumours	*Malignant Tumours*
1. They develop slowly.	They grow rapidly.
2. Remain localised and encapsulated.	Do not remain localised, but infiltrate into the neighbouring tissues and there is no tendency for encapsulation.
3. Are not harmful ; the only harm they can do is by pressure upon other organs, tissues and nerves.	Are greatly harmful, because they take away all the blood and nutrition at the expense of the person who grows weaker and emaciated while the tumour enlarges.
4. The proportion and normal disposition of various tissues remain intact with no tendency to disorganise the tissues.	There is a tendency to disorganise the tissues by growth of cells into the neighbouring tissues.
5. There is no secondary growth or metastasis.	There is a tendency to secondary growth and metastasis. The cells of malignant tumours are transported to other parts of the body through lymphatics and blood stream where they grow and form new secondary growths.
6. When they are excised or operated, there is no tendency to recur.	Even after operation, there is a tendency to recur.
7. Infections, ulcerations, necrosis and haemorrhages are not common.	Infections, ulcerations, necrosis and haemorrhages are very common.
8. The tissues are of normal type.	The cells are not of normal type and resemble the embryonic type.

9. The cells do not contain nuclei ; they are of adult type.	The cells show mitotic division having multiple nuclei.
10. The blood vessels are few but well formed.	There are numerous blood vessels and the tumour contains a large supply of blood.
11. There is a basement membrane.	The basement membrane is absent.

Sarcoma	*Carcinoma*
1. Mesoblastic origin.	Hypo or epiblastic origin.
2. Stroma surrounds individual cells.	Storma surrounds masses of cells.
3. Embryonic, round or spindle shaped cells.	Cells are epithelial in nature, columnar, cubical, spheroidal or flattened.
4. The blood vessels are in contact with the cells of the tumour and may be formed by modification of these cells ; haemorrhage is common.	The blood vassels are entirely contained in the stroma.
5. The spread is through blood stream.	The spread is through lymphatics and blood stream.
6. It destroys the tissue by pressure withont producing any fibrous reaction.	Fibrous tissue reaction is persent surrounding carcinoma.
7. New young capillaries develop for the nutrition.	No new vessels form in cancer mass. they appear in the fibrous tissue stroma.
8. No alveolar arrangment, as there is no fibrous tissue reaction.	Alveolar arrangement is there, on account of fibrous tissue reaction.
9. Great malignancy due to the blood vessels.	Invades the local tissue and ultimately the lymphatics, then the adjacent glands and finally the blood stream.

CYSTS

CYST means a space, sac or cavity containing the fluid of serous or mucoid character of colourless or a yellow tint or it may be brownish owing to the admixture of altered blood; degenerated epithelium may also be present. It is lined by epithelium or endothelium and arises from the dilatation of the pre-existing tubules, ducts or cavities.

Classification

The cysts are of two varieties :—

1. Congenital cysts, and
2. Acquired cysts.

Congenital Cysts or Dermoid Cysts : These are found in the middle line of the chest and neck at the outer or inner angle of the orbit ; e.g., meningocele, encephalocele and spina bifida. These types of cysts develop due to some congenital defect in the body.

Acquired Cysts : They develop in the normal organs due to the development of some sort of abnormality in them. They are further classified into the following :—

1. *Retention Cysts* : They occur due to the retention of the secretions in certain ducts, glands or cavities of the body on account of some sort of obstruction in their outflow; e.g., in the kidneys, uterine tubes, salivary glands, pancreas, gall-bladder, etc.
2. *Distension and Exudation Cysts* :—They develop due to the dilatation of the ducts or glandular structures, which, later on, are filled with excessive secretory material ; e.g., thyroid, pituitary and ovaries.
3. *Implanation and Parasitic Cysts* :—This type of cysts develops on account of presence of some parasite ; e.g.. Hydatid cyst due to Taenia echinococcus.

——

TUMOURS OF THE UTERUS

CHAPTER XXXXII

FIBROMYOMA

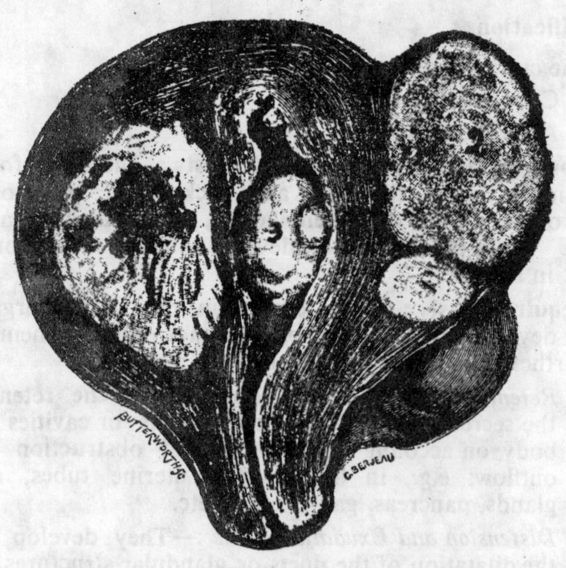

Submucous, Intramural and Subserous Fibroids.

It is the benign growth of the uterus originating from the fibrous and muscular tissues of the uterus. It is encapsulated; therefore, there is no wild growth. It is an innocent growth, so, it is called benign.

Aetiology :

No definite cause is known; but according to homoeopathy, it is sycotic in nature.

1. **Infertility :** Probably tumours of the uterus are caused by infertility, and vice-versa.
2. **Hypersecretion of Oestrin :** Oestrin and Progesterone are the secretions of the ovaries. Oestrin controls the activities of uterus and the breasts. Its action is proliferation, regeneration and growth; and excessive growth might prove a cause in the development of fibroids.
3. **Heredity :** Heredity is an important factor in the causation of fibroids. Tuberculosis, asthma, tumours, paralysis, piles, heart diseases are all hereditary and have a sycotic base.

As a matter of fact, nothing certain is known of the aetiology except the constant irritition either due to injury or other activities, causes, does excite the tissues to neoplastic.

It is most common in the body of the uterus (in about 92% cases). In the body there are a number of growths, whereas in the cervix it is single.

Common age of occurence

It is 30-45 years. Before 20 years of age, there are no chances of the tumour formation. Similarly after menopause, these fibroids are rare.

Types of Uterine Fibromyoma :

1. Interstitial ... in about 50% cases.
2. Submucous ... in about 30% cases.
3. Subserous ... in about 20% cases.

Interstitial : means growing the tissue; it grows within the musuclar wall.

Subserous or Subperitoneal : If it protrudes outside carrying with it the peritoneal wall, it is called subserous; it is also called sub-peritoneal, i. e., protruding towards the serous coat.

Submucous : And, if it starts protruding towards inside of the cavtiy carrying with it the endometrium, the mucous lining, it is called submucous. Submucous variety is further classified into :—

(i) Sessile, and

(ii) Pendeculated.

Sessile : means growing directly from the stem ; and

Pedenculated : means hanging from a supporting part; that is also called a polypus.

Future Fate of Submucous Fibroid

1. It may become pedenculated; i. e., the formation of a polypus.
2. Chances of infection.
3. It may turn in to a milgnant condition.
4. It may cause inversion of the uterus during the process of contraction.
5. Changes in the uterus and adenexes, supporting structures and associated lesions :
   (i) Enlargement of the cavity in submucous and interstitial varieties.
   (ii) Hypertrophy of the muscles of uterus.
   (iii) Ovaries are also hypertrophied and cystic: it may be due to over production of oestrin.
   (iv) Fallopian tubes : chronic inflammatory lesion may be present, which may be due to secondary infection.
   (v) Ureters are compressed, especially in the subserous variety ; so, there may be obstruction in the flow of the urine causing hydronephrotic condition of the kidneys.

The endometrium is thickened due to hyperaemia caused by the tumour or excessive ovarian secretion. There is chronic congestion ; and, this gives rise to leucorrhoea and also menorrhagia. The uterine cavity is enlarged and the position of uterus is distorted to that side.

Pathology

Naked eye appearance : The tumour is pale and silk like and there is whorld derangement of interlacing fibres. If the capsule is cut, the tumoūr protrudes convexly.

Microscopic picture : It consists of muscular and white fibrous tissue. The blood vessels vary depending upon the hardness or softness of the tumour. The capsule also contains the blood vessels. The ovaries are cystic in nature in about 25% of cases and the tubes are often the seat of chronic inflammation.

Associated lesions with uterine fibroids

1. *Endometeriosis* :-- It means a growth of endometrium like tissue, somewhere else (in ovaries or pelvis or peritoneum) which will undergo the same cyclical changes as is with the endometrium itself, due to hypersecretion of oestrin.
2. *Adeno-Carcinoma* may also co-exist.
3. *Associated genital prolapse*
4. *Ovarian tumours*
5. *Polycythaemia* : It means the persistent increase of RBCs.
6. *High Blood Pressure* : Once fibroids are removed, blood pressure will also come down.

Results of Fibromyoma

1. Degeneration : It may be destroyed [by degeneration of any variety or it may become necrosed.

(i) *Atrophy* : It may atrophy during menopause or sometimes by the application of deep X-rays or oophorectomy.

(ii) *Hyaline Degeneration* : It may occur due to malnutrition. (Hyaline means transparent).

(iii) *Cystic Degeneration* : Cyst contains thick fluid as a result of liquefaction of hyaline tissue.

(iv) *Fatty Degeneration* : Here, the appearance will be yellow.

(v) *Calcareal Degeneration* : Calcareal deposits (mostly lime) are accumulated, as a result of which degeneration starts.

(vi) *Necrosis* : It is due to the lack of supply of blood.

(vii) *Necrobiosis* : It is partial necrosis; i. e., still there is life in it and the colour is reddish.

2. Infection :—Infection may occur at the site of the tumour, esp. with the submucous variety; such as Pelvic cellulitis.

3. Malignant Change :— It may undergo a malignant change, especially with a recurring polypus.

Symptoms :

History of amenorrhoea is altogether absent.

1. Persistent and progressive menorrhagia.
2. Metrorrhagia.
3. Leucorrhoea.
4. Dysmenorrhoea.
5. Palpable mass per abdomen.
6. Pressure symptoms (in subserous variety); such as pelvic pain, constipation, venous obstruction, oedema of legs and frequency of micturition.
7. Anaemia due to loss of blood through menorrhagia and metrorrhagia.
8. Secondary symptoms may turn to malignancy.
9. Hyperacidity of stomach is a very common symptom.

Signs :

1. Pallor, due to anaemia.
2. High blood pressure, in some cases.
3. Per abdomen, a swelling is felt in the hypogastrium.
4. This swelling is firm and mobile.
5. It has well defined margins.
6. On auscultation. we can hear the uterine soufle (soufle is a a murmuring sound caused by the gush of blood to the broad ligaments—the uterine vessels).
7. On P.V. examination—in submucous variety, pelvic mass can be felt arising from the uterus.
8. Sterility is common, which is due to the accompanying salpingitis or endometritis. If pregnancy takes place, abortion or necrobiosis may result.

Differential Diagnosis :

1. **Pregnancy** : History of amenorrhoea is important alongwith other signs and symptoms of pregnancy. Biological tests for pregnancy are positive.

2. **Metropathia haemorrhogica** : It is a functional uterine bleeding due to hyperplasia of the endometrium as a result of excessive secretion.

3. **Ovarian cyst** :—Here, menorrhagia is not there.

4. **Full bladder** :—History of retention of urine is there and the urine can be passed by the catheter.

5. **Hydatidiform mole** : History of amenorrhoea is present.

6. **Sub-Involution of ut erus after delivery** : Uterus is is more or less regular in outline; and it never enlarges more than the size of 3-4 months pregnancy.

Causes of death in fibroids, if left untreated :

1. Haemorrhage and severe anaemia.
2. Intraperitoneal haemorrhage due to the rupture of sub-serous veins.
3. Peritonitis due to suppuration of fibroids; and
4. Malignancy.

Complications :

1. **Infection** : It may come through the vagina or tubes of from the inflamed neighbouring parts; or the inflammation may develop in the endometrium; i.e., auto-infection.

Suppuration is rare and the sloughing occurs due to necrosis.

2. **Adhesions** : Although rare, they may occur due to appendicitis or salpingitis.

3. **Axial rotation** : Tumour, by its own weight, rotates. It may occur with sub-peritoneal variety which has long stalk. If the tumour becomes congested and adhesions are formed, it may cause pain and sometimes rise of temperature.

4. **Malignant changes** : They may also take place; e.g., endothelioma, carcinoma and sarcoma.

Sure Method of diagnosing malignancy is by Biopsy and microscopic examination. Yet, we can suspect it in the presence of the following points :—

(i) If the tumour grows much after menopause.

(ii) Return of bleeding after menopause.

(iii) When the tumour becomes soft and starts growing rapidly.

(iv) Local pain over the tumour.

(v) Wasting of the body without any apparent cause.

(vi) Recurrence of polypi.

Uterine Fibroid	*Ovarian Cyst*
1. Solid and hard.	Cystic feeling.
2. Cervix usually continuous.	Neither continuous nor moves with the tumour.
3. Sound in the uterus moves the tumour mass.	No movement.
4. Uterine cavity is enlarged.	No enlargement.
5. Uterine soufle may be heard.	Not present.
6. Menorrhagia.	No menorrhagia.

Treatment :

Treatment is mostly symptomatic. Many authorities consider that the fibroids should be left alone; but, extra modern practitioners recommend radiotherapy and operation.

Radiotherapy undoubtedly helps to stop bleeding; but, it may be dangerous to produce necrosis and other things.

Three types of operations are carried out :—

(i) Supra-vaginal hysterectomy.

(ii) Pan-hysterectomy.

(iii) Myomectomy.

1. Bed rest.
2. Calcium with vit. C and K.

3. Hormonal treatment in modern system.
4. If there is excessive and severe anaemia, blood-transfusion.
5. Then, suitable *homoeopathic remedies* :–

All Calcarea group, Aur. met., Aur, mur., Aur, mur natronatum, Lach., Lil. tig, Phos., Sil., Thuja, Puls.

For bleeding :

Bell., Erigeron., Ipec., Millef., Sab., Trillium, Vib. op., Ustilago, Ham. China, Fer. Phos., Secalc C., and Platina (Calc. Carb., China, Ustilago and Sabina—for profuse bleeding, so much so that blood transfusion becomes necessary.)

CHAPTER XLII
POLYPUS OF THF UTERUS

POLYPUS of uterus is a mass of the new formation that tends to grow or persist without fulfilling any physiological function and with no typical termination.

It is benign to start with, but can become malignant in unfavourable cases. Occasionally, when the fibromyoma becomes pedenculated, then a fibroid polypus of the uterus may develop and that may project through the os into the vagina where it may undergo strangulation or torsion and may slough away or become acutely inflamed.

The polypi may be of different varieties :

1. Fibroid type.
2. Placental type.
3. Mucous polypi in the endometrium.
4. Sarcomatous polypi.

These polypi may develop outside the uterus also, e. g., in the tubes, ovaries, round ligaments and recto-vaginal connective tissue.

There is a special type also, named Intermittent polypus which appears at the os only during menstruation owing to slight cervical dilatation at that time. Uterine contractions forcing it down, it disappears between the periods.

Dangers of Polyi :

1. Bleeding.
2. Leucorrhoea.
3. Malignancy.

Therefore, all polypi should be examined under the microscope for malignancy.

Treatment :

Removal of the polypus is the rule; and after that suitable remedies should be given symptomatically.

——

CHAPTER XLIII

CARCINOMA OF THE UTERUS

CARCINOMA of the uterus is fairly common and accounts for over 30% of deaths from this disease. It is usually uncomon before the age of 30 years (exceptions are, however, there). It commonly occurs after 50 years of age (50–65 years) and in multipara mostly. It has no relation with the child bearing. It is usually associated with ulceration or erosion of the cervix to start with.

The growth is merely always adeno-carcinomatous and occasionally squamous-cell epithelioma.

The extension occurs in the parametrium. It may extend down to the cervix or the spread takes place by the lymphatics. Secondary growths in the liver, lungs and pleura are more common than cervical cancer.

Symptoms :

1. Bleeding after menopause is a classical symptom; e. g., 1 or 2 years after the cessation of menses. At first, it is excessive menorrhagia ; then it turns into metrorrhagia. It may also occur while straining at stools and during coitus. Discharges are very foul and offensive containing muco-pus and cancerous debris.

2. Pain appears late indicating its extension beyond the uterus. Pain unfortunately is not an early symptom, hence the cancer is diagnosed late. Sometimes, it is so late that the tumour is advanced a great deal. Pain, when felt, is of gnawing or boring character. There may also be sympathetic or referred pain in the back, breasts and legs.

3. Discharge may be absent; but, when present, is always watery.

4. Secondary growth in the peritoneum is marked by multiple masses, abdominal distension and ascites.

Other important symptoms are :

5. Wasting : loss of flesh.

6. Debility : general weakness, and

7. Cachexia : a condition occuring due to the absorption of toxins causing debility, weakness, etc.

Physical Signs :

1. In ulcerating growths, the uterus is not enlarged; and when no ulceration is present, it is enlarged, but never larger than three months pregnancy size.

2. The uterus does not become fixed, until very late.

Differential Diagnosis :

1. Post menopausal bleeding can occur in many conditions, but they are all unimportant; e.g.,
   (i) Senile endometritis.
   (ii) Senile vaginitis.
2. Mucous polypus and fibroid.
3. Biopsy.
   Remember, continuous bleeding is always abnormal. Whatever be the age and cause , we must exclude the cancerous condition.

Treatment :

The basic principle of treating cancer is an excision of entire uterus with the surrounding tissues. However, this method is indicated in the initial stages (i.e. first and second); in other cases, surgical operation is not indicated, only X-ray and radium therapy may help to some extent. However, after the growth has extended and metastasis has taken place, it is not possible to control the disease.

Use of Stilboestrol or other Oestrin preparations are prescribed to relieve menopausal symptoms, i.e , withdrawal bleeding.

And, then, the homoeopathic remedies to be given on the **basis of symptomatology** :—

Cadmium salts, Calcareas, Ars. iod., Carbo. an., Hydras., Kreosote, Puls., Kali iod., Kali C., Lach., Palladium, Teucrium, Alumen, Thuja, Medo., Sil., Nux v., Ipec., Bufo., Apis, Aur. m. nat., Lil. tig., Phos., Ustilago, Natm.; Terebinth, Erigeron, Millef., Tril., Vib. op., Ham., China, Ferrum Phos., Bell., Secaleand Platina.

——

CHAPTER XLIV

SARCOMA OF THE UTERVS

SARCOMA is another variety of malignant tumours of the uterus. It is, of course, of rare occurance. If ever it occurs, the body of uterus is commonly involved.

Age incidence is the same, i.e., 45–55 years. Metastasis occurs early to the lungs through the blood stream and to the peritoneum directly.

Aetiology

It is the same as in other malignant tumours of the uterus.

Signs and Symptoms :

As pointed out earlier, in case of sarcomatous affections, pain is the first sign. Then, there is discharge and thereafter bleeding. Per abdomen, we can feel the bulge as the uterus gets enlarged. We find cachexia, loss of weight, ascites and distension of veins over the abdomen also.

Differential Diagnosis :

1. Fibromyoma.
2. Corcinoma.

Fibromyoma is an affection of earlier life than cancer.

And, carinoma is differentiated by the symptoms : such as, bleeding, discharge and lastly the pain; whereas, in sarcoma, there is pain first, then discharge and then bleeding.

Treatment :

Basic principle is the removal of the uterus in all the malignant conditions of the uterus. But, in some cases, deep X-ray and radium therapy help to some extent. Alongwith it, *homoeopathic remedies* can also be given with results.

Bufo., Apis, Calcareas, Aur. m· nat., Cadm. salts, China, Ferr. Phos., Ham , Kali iod., Kreosote, Lil. Tig., Lach., Puls., Thuja, Ustilago, Vib. op.

TUMOURS OF THE CERVIX

CHAPTER XLV

FIBROID

1. It is found mostly on the posterior wall of the cervix.
2. It has a uniform outline and is usually single as the space for its growth is very limited.
3. Uterine body is elevated, but not enlarged.
4. Cervical canal in enlarged and laterally expanded.
5. External os is expanded to form a slit owing to the tumour tending to become partially submucous.
6. External os is drawn up and may be displaced upwards and laterally.
7. Uterine vessels are displaced as also the ureters which may be stretched over the capsule.
8. Large growth, the lymphatics and vessels of the broad ligament are enormously dilated and may give rise to much bleeding at the time of operation.

Clinical features :

Most important are the pressure symptoms; e.g.,

1. Retention of urine.
2. Bleeding is never a sign of the uncomplicated and purely cervical fibroid.

——

CHAPTER XLVII

POLYPUS OF THE CERVIX

It is a pedenculated tumour arising from the mucous membrane of the cervix. Usually, it is benign, but may become malignant. No definite cause has been attributed to its occurance; but, it has been agreed that it is due to the hereditary tendency (with sycosis at the root) and hypersecretion of oestrin whose action is proliferation, regeneration and growth.

Common age of occurance is 30 to 45 years; before 20 years, there are no chances; similarly, after menopaus, eits occurance rare.

Signs and Symptoms

1. Bleeding is an important symptom.
2. Leucorrhoea.
3. A mass, protruding out of external os intc the vagina can be felt through P.V. examination.

Treatment

Treatment is mostly symptomatic. Many authorities consider that the fibroid should be left alone; but extra modern practitioners recommend radio herapy and operation.

Radiotherapy, undoubtedly, helps to stop bleeding; but, may be dangerous to produce necrosis and other things.

Homoeopathic remedies :

Aurum iod., Aurum mur., Calc, carb., Calc. iod., Calendula, Conium, Fraxinus americana, Hydrocotyle, Iodium. Kali iod., Lach., Nitric acid, Phos., Sabina, Thlaspi bur., Thuja and Thyroidinum.

— —

CHAPTER XLVII
CARCINOMA OF THE CERVIX

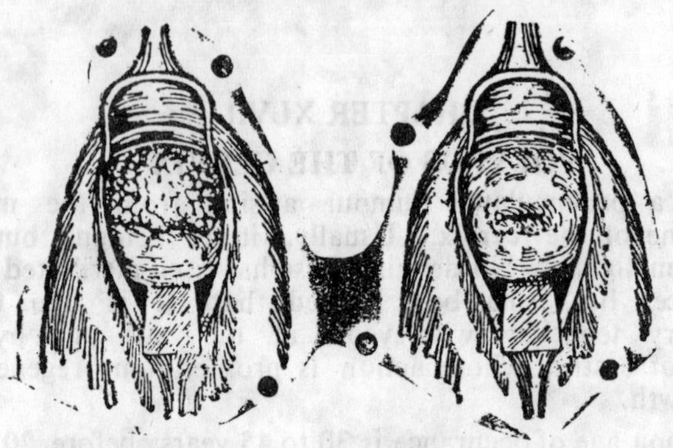

Healthy Uterus   Cancer of the posterior cervical lip.

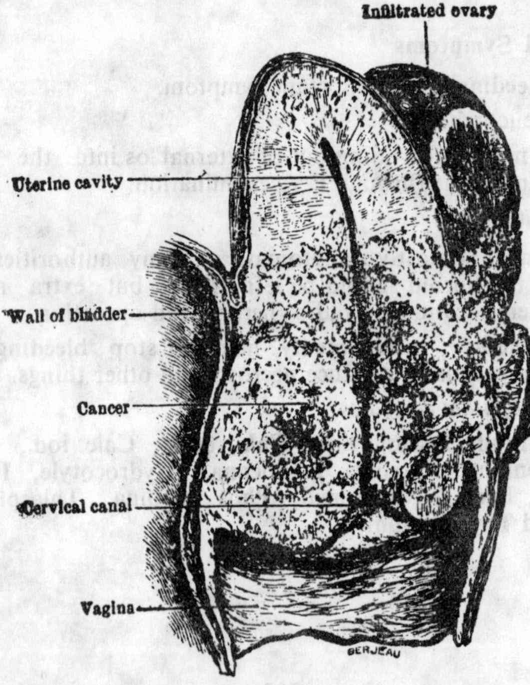

Infiltrated ovary

Uterine cavity

Wall of bladder

Cancer

Cervical canal

Vagina

BERJEAU

Advanced carcinoma of the cervix

1. Either, it begins on the surface of the cervix around the os where the growth is mostly of the squamous cells.

2. Or, it may also grow in the cervical canal. Here, the growth is adenomatous in character arising from the cervical glands.

Cervical irritation may predispose to carcinoma of the cervix.

The spread is by lymphatic permeation. Metastasis to distant organs may also be through blood stream; but, it is uncommon.

Infiltration will extend into the parametrium, inter-iliac and common iliac glands.

Aetiology

1. Prolonged use of pessaries and chemical contraceptives.
2. Excessive oestrin secretion.
3. Congenital erosion.
4. Excessive alkalinity of vaginal secretions.
5. Tendency to malignancy.

Symptoms :

1. Irregular bleeding brought on at the time of examination, douching, intercourse or touch; later, it becomes continuous with varying amount. It may be mistaken for irregular menses of the climacteric.

2. Watery discharge : it may become offensive when infection is present.

3. Pain : indicating extension of the condition to the peritoneum and other surrounding structures.

4. Dysuria and frequency of micturition.

5. Incontinence of urine or stool, dribbling, ulceration extending to the bladder.

6. Cachexia : rapid loss of weight, debility, etc.

Physical signs :

Early cases :

1. A small nodule or small ulcer like erosion is seen.
2. Frequent bleeding on slightest touch.

B-Class

1. A warty or cowliflower like growth.
2. A deep crater shaped ulcer with hard, high and developed margins.
3. Free bleeding on P.V. examination, intercourse and touch.
4. Thin watery and blood mixed offensive discharge offensiveness comes later on).

Carcinoma—Bleeding, discharge, then pain.

Sarcoma—Pain, discharge, then bleeding.

Endocarcinoma of cervical canal

In early cases, there is bleeding and no other abnormality. Later when developed : the cervix is enlarged, hard and barrel shaped; and when thegrowth breaks down and is sloughed, a deep ulcer with hard indurated edges is felt.

Differential Diagnosis :

1. Cervical erosion : Ulceration, age (younger group), it does not bleed on touch.
2. Mucous polypus : Felt as coming from the os.
3. Tuberculosis of cervix : Here, the history of tuberculosis is important. Biopsy should be done.
4. Carcinoma of body of uterus.

Carcinoma of the Cervix	*Carcinoma of body of Uterus*
1. Very common (15 : 1 ratio)	Much more rare.
2. Occurs mostly in parous women, with large family	Common in nullipara and in women with small family.
3. Occurs between the age of 45 to 55 years.	Occurs between 50 to 60 years of age.
4. Very malignant.	Less malignant.
5. Uterine body not enlarged	Body is uniformly enlarged.
6. Fibro-muscular wall involved early.	Involved late.
7. Squamous cell type common.	Columnar cell type common.

Carcinoma of the Cervix	Carcinoma of body of Uterus
8. Ulceration is common.	Ulceration is not common.
9. Prognosis is bad, if not treated early.	Good unless very advanced.
10. Iliac & sacral lymphatic glands involved first.	Lumbar and inguinal glands first involved; iliac and sacral glands are involved late.
11. Werth-heim operation is indicated.	Pan-hysterectomy.
12. Only operable early, in 1-6 months time.	Operable after much longer time.
13. Death: $1\frac{1}{2}$ years from onset, if left alone and untreated.	Death : 2-4 years from onset of symptoms.

Death is due to

1. Uraemic conditions; blockage or infection.
2. Haemorrhage and exhaustion, and
3. Secondary growth.

Stages of Cancer :

First stage : The growth is limited to the cervix and the uterus is mobile.

Second stage : The lesion spreads to one or two fornices without infiltration of parametrium; but the uterus retains some mobility.

Third stage : There is nodular infiltration of the parametrium on one or both sides extending to the walls of the pelvis with limited mobility of the uterus or there will be massive infiltration of the parametrium (cellular tissue) with fixation of the uterus. There may also be superficial ulceration of the vagina. There is metastasis in the pelvic glands or lower part of the vagina.

Fourth stage : When the fourth stage comes, the following findings would be there :

(i) Massive infiltration on both sides, parametrium extending to the pelvic walls.

(ii) Invasion of the bladder and rectum.

(iii) Infiltration of the vaginal walls, wholly or partially.

(iv) Metastasis to remote places.

Course and Complications :

The discharges assume a yellowish, brownish or bloody colour; and when decomposition of tissues begins, they become brownish. Ulceration causes secondary infection and a foetid smell comes out. The cervix uteri is enlarged and tuberous; and the tumour extends to adjacent vaginal canal and easily bleeds when touched with a finger. The cervix looks like a cauliflower. Subsequently, the process extends to the parametric connective tissues and involves the nerve fibres, causing excruciating pains. The growth extends to the adjacent organs-urinary bladder and rectum ; fistula appears and metastasis in distant organs may occur. A progressive cachexia develops due to general toxaemia and death takes place within 12—18 months.

Treatment :

The basic principle of treating cancer is an excision of the entire uterus with the surrounding tissues. However, this method is indicated in cases of incipient cancer and in first and second stages. In all other cases, surgical operation is not indicated.

Only X-ray and radium therapy may help somewhat ; that means, when the cervix is mobile, i. e. in stage 1 & 2, life can be extended for 5-10 years.

However, after the growth has extended and metastasis has teken place, i. e., in stage 3 & 4, it is not possible to control the condition.

Mostly, the treatment in such cases, is symptomatic with suitable *homoeopathic remedies* :

Ars., Ars. iod., Nit. acid, Arg. nit, Calcareas, Carbo an., Carbolic acid, Conium, Phos., Hydras., Kreosote, Lach., Merc., Phos., Secale, Sepia, Thuja and Cadm. Salts.

—

TUMOURS OF THE UTERUS AND CERVIX

THERAPEUTIC HINTS

Arsenic : Great exhaustion; restlessness and fits of angu with terrible, sharp, burning pains; all worse about midnight; acrid, corroding and burning discharges, watery, light or dark coloured, often very offensive.

Aurum mur : Stinging, cutting pressive pains in the uterine region; very offensive discharges ; belching up of wind; craves nothing but sour things.

Belladonna : Painful bearing down in the pelvis, as though everything would fall out of the genitals ; a similar pain in the back; frequent, transient stitches in the region of the womb; haemorrhages from the womb, profuse, often very offenisve.

Calc. carb : Burning soreness in the genital organs; aching in the vagina ; profuse menstruation ; flow of blood between the monthly periods; cold feeling on the top of the head; great sensitiveness to cold air and liability to catch cold; scrofulous diathesis. Uterine polypi; with sterility ; fair, fat and flabby patient.

Carbo animalis : Burning in the abdomen, extending into the thighs ; labour like pain in the pelvis and small of the back extending into the thighs, with discharge of slimy, discoloured; blood; irregular menses; uterus swollen and hard; cachetic oppearance of the face; earthy colour of the skin; great weakness.

Carbo veg : Paroxysmal spell of burning in the uterin region ; varicose veins on the external organs ; cold knees in bed.

Conium : Stitching pain in the womb, accompanied by such symptoms as accompany pregnancy ; nausea and vomiting; craving for sour or salty things; pain and swelling of the mammae during the menses ; dejection of spirits, etc.

Graphites : Cauliflower excrescence ; burning, stitching pains, like electric shocks, through the womb, extending into the thighs ; great heaviness in the abdomen when standing, with increased pains and faintness ; menses only every six weeks, with a discharge of black, clotted, offensive blood and an increase of all the sufferings; constipation; earthy colour of the face; frequent chilliness ; and despondings.

Iodium : Cutting in the abdomen, with pains in the loins and small of the back; uterine haemorrhage at every stool ; indurations of the uterus ; painfulness and feeling of heaviness in both mammae; they hang down, relaxed and lose their fat ; dwindling and falling away of the mammae ; the patient feels worse from external warmth; after abuse of mercury.

Kreosote : Cauliflower excrescence ; awful burning as of red hot coal in the pelvis, with discharge of clots of blood having a foul smell; bearing down and sense of weight in the pelvis, drawing pains in the small of the back and uterine region, extending to the thighs, intermingled with stitching pains ; the vagina is swollen and burning hot ; long standing leucorrhoea, becoming more and more watery, acrid, bloody and ichorous all the time; frequent haemorrhages from the womb; dwindling and falling away of the mammae, with small, hard, painful lumps in them, wretched complexion ; great debility ; sleeplessness.

Lachesis : Pain in the parts as if swollen, they do not bear contact, and have to be relieved of all pressure; coughing or sneezing causes stitching pains in the affected parts; tenacious and acrid menstrual flow with labour like pains; discharge of a few drops of blood from the nose before menses, which are scanty and delaying; especially indicated during the climacteric period with frequent uterine haemorrhages.

Lycopodium : Drawing in the groins ; burning and gnawing; chronic dryness of the vagina; pressing through the vagina on stooping; discharge of wind through the vagina; pain in the small of the back, extending down to the feet; incarcerated flatulence, with rumbling in the left hypochondriac region; red, sandy sediment in the urine; jerking of single limbs awake or asleep; feels worse in general from 4 to 8 O' clock in the evening.

Magnesia mur : Scirrhous induration of the womb ; uterine spasms extending to the thighs and occasioning leuccorrhoea; discharge of black clots of menstrual blood, more when sitting than when walking; large, hard, difficult stools which crumble off as they are expelled.

Merc Sol: Syphilitic taint; prolapse of the vagina; swelling of inguinal glands.

Murex purp: A lively, affectionate disposition has turned to melancholy from the effects of the disease; frequent, profuse menstruation, and strong sexual desire; in the region of the cervix, or a feeling as though something was pressing on a sore spot in the pelvis; with pain in the right side of the uterus going into the abdomen or thorax; watery greenish leucorrhoea, irritating the parts; dragging and relaxation in the perineum; pains in the hips, loins, and down the thighs, worse from exertion.

Nitric acid: Irregular menstruation in shorter or longer intervals; during the intervals a profuse, discoloured, brownish and offensive leucorrhoea; great debility, nervousness, and depression of spirits; haemorrhoidal tendency; great pain in the rectum after stools, lasting for hours, even worse after a dierrhoeic evacuation; the urine is very offensive. During a ride in the carriage they feel much better.

Natrum carb.: Induration of the neck of the womb; the os uteri is out of shape; pressing in the hypogastrium towards the genital organs, as if everything would come out; metrorrhagia; putrid leucorrhoea; headache in the sun and from mental labour; she gets nervous from playing on the piano, and feels great anxiety during a thunder storm.

Phosphorus: Frequent and profuse metrorrhagia, pouring out freely and then ceasing for a short time; heat in the back; chlorotic appearance; instead of menses; watery, slimy or acrid discharge, causing blisters.

Phytolacca: Menses too frequent and too copious; mammae painful; sterility; constipation; syphilitic taint.

Rhus tox.: Great soreness in vagina preventing an embrace; the menstrual flow, being profuse, protracted, and of light colour, causes biting pain in the vulva.

Sepia: Induration colli uteri or vaginae; painful stiffness in the uterus; pressing from above downwards, oppressing the breathing; must cross her thighs, in order to get relief; pot-belliedness; yellow saddle across the bridge of the nose; feels worse while riding in a carriage. Menses scanty; aversion to coitus; sad, indifferent.

Silicea : She feels nauseated during an embrace; diarrhoea or else great costiveness before the menses, increased menses, with repeated paroxysms of icy coldness over the whole body at the time of their appearance; induration of the mammae; most of the symptoms make their appearance about new moon. Cysts in the vagina, as large as a pea or an orange, projecting from the vagina.

Tarentula : Cancerous ulcer of os, induration of neck and fundus, chronic vaginitis with granulations.

Thuja : Cauliflower excrescences ; polypus on the cervix, prolapsus uteri, faulty menses; pain in the uterine region with scanty and burning urine; simple tumours. Bleeding fungi; epithelial variety of cancer; also useful in sarcoma and papilloma.

Hydrastis : Of undoubted and special value in epithelioma and uterine cancer. Simple glandular tumours of the breast; it relieves the pain, retards the growth and improves the patient generally. Dyspeptic symptoms. One of the best known remedies for cancer. Worn jaded look, sallow complexion; loss of appetite, hidebound state of the skin, low spirits, constipation.

Cuprum acet : Relieves the distressing vomitting in carcinoma.

Radium brom. : A remedy for pre-cancerous stage; with aching pains, itching over the body, pains resembling a chronic arthritis. Apprehension; mentally tired and irritable patient. Pimples on the skin and spots which itch and burn. Restlessness, heat in stomach, flatulence and constipation.

Carbolic acid : A valuable internal remedy in cancer. Pustules about the vulva containing bloody pus. Agonizing backache across loins, with dragging down the thighs. Pain in left ovary, worse walking in open air. Erosion of cervix with foetid, acrid discharge.

Cedron : For lancinating pains of cancers.

Pulsatilla : An excellent remedy for fibroid tumours, especially in the uterine wall near the fundus.

Kali Iod. : Fibroid tumour of the uterus. This remedy may be tried if Pulsatilla fails. Womb packed with fibroid tumours; tired sleepy feeling down the limbs, hot burning feet, though sometimes immense shivering all over.

Kali carb. : Cancer of the uterus with severe pain from hip to knee, especially right side. Pain in leg is characteristic of this remedy.

Palladium : Ovarian tumours.

Teucrium : Polypus in vagina.

Alumen : Ovarian tumour with obstinate constipation.

Nux Vomica and Ipecac. : Uterine fibroma in hydrogenoid constitutions ; as such, the symptoms are worse in wet weather and by water.

Bufo : Cancer with red streaks.

Cadimum salts : (Cadmium met., Cadm. iod., Cadm. phos. & Cadm. sulph.) :

For the cancer of the uterus after radium treatment has failed. They may be tried with good results.

Aurum mur natronatum : Uterine tumours with high blood pressure. Indurated cervix. Chronic metritis and prolapsus. Uterus fills up the whole of the pelvis. Ulceration of the neck of the womb and vagina. Leucorrhoea, with spasmodic contraction of vagina. Ovaries are indurated. Ovarian dropsy. Sub-involution. Ossified uterus.

Calarea fluor. : A routine tissue remedy in the treatment of the tumours. The tumours are hard to feel : often associated with displacements of the uterus. Dragging pain in the region of the uterus and thighs, bearing down of the uterus. Varicose veins of the vulva. Uterine fibroids. Knots, kernels, hardened glands in the breasts.

—

TUMOURS OF OVARIES

CHAPTER XLVIII

BENIGN

Benign tumours are of different types according to their origin :—

1. Epithelial tissue tumour.
2. Connective tissue tumour.
3. Mixed tumour.
4. Endothelial tumour.

1. Epithelial tissue tumours : They are of different varieties :

(i) Benign type of cyst or multilocular cyst.

(ii) Pesudo-membranous (mucinous) cyst-adenoma.

(iii) Palilomatous cyst.

(iv) Granulomatous cyst.

2. Connective tissue tumours : Connective tissue tumours are.

(i) Fibroma, and

(ii) Fibromyoma.

3. Mixed tumours : Cystic teratoma or dermoid cyst.

4. Endothelial tumours : Endometrioma.

Papilomatous Cyst	*Pseudo-Muccinous Cyst*
1. Rare occurrence : 10%	Very common.
2. Usually bilateral.	Usually unilateral.
3. It is ligamentous (between the ligaments).	Pedenculated.
4. Often displaces the uterus upwards.	Slight displacement.

Papilomatous Cyst	Pseudo-Muccinous Cyst
5. Causes elongation of supra-vaginal cervix.	No elongation of cervix.
6. Unilocular.	Multilocular.
7. Fluid is serous.	Fluid is pseudo-mucinous.
8. Size is small, not bigger than a melon.	Very large size.
9. Epithelium may be columnar or ciliated.	Always columnar.
10. Metastasis on rupture.	No metastasis.
11. Very apt to become malignant.	Not so malignant.

CHAPTER XLIX

MALIGNANT TUMOURS OF THE OVARIES

Malignant tumours of the ovaries may be—

1. Primary, or
2. Secondary.

1. Primary malignant tumours : These are of three varieties :

(i) Malignant pailomatous cyst adenoma.

(ii) Malignant pseudo-mucinous cyst adenoma.

(iii) Solid carcinoma.

2. Secondary malignant tumours : These tumours are metastatic from the uterus, stomach, intestines and breasts. They are of following types :—

(i) *Connective tissue tumours* :

(a) Sarcoma.

(b) Endothelioma.

(c) Perithelioma.

(ii) *Mixed type of tumours* : Solid teratoma : (Tera means three and toma means layers. All the three layers of embryo are there and covered by the skin).

— —

CHAPTER L

CYSTS OF THE OVARIES

Ovarian tumours are mostly the cystic tumours. They are mostly benign tumours, but may become malignant in unfavourable conditions. Cysts are quite common in old age.

A CYST is a rounded cavity with distinct lining of the membrane containing the fluid or semi-solid material.

1. Follicular Cyst :

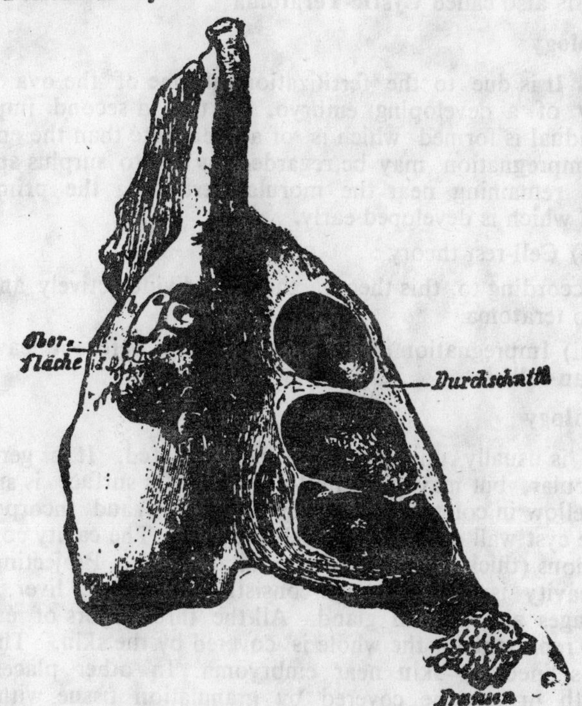

Ovary with Dropsical Follicles. (Natural size.) a, b, three cysts ; c.d.e., Obreflache, surface of the ovary ; Durchschnitt, section ; Fransen, fimbriae.

It is due to the non-rupture of a graffian follicle. Degeneration may occur in the ovum (ovaries)—membrane granulosa increasing the liquor-follicle with cystic distension.

2. Lutein Cyst :

There is accumulation of fluid in thè corpus luteum. There may be no symptoms or there may be irregular bleeding.

3. Dermoid Cyst :

It is also called **Cystic-Teratoma**

Aetiology

(i) It is due to the fertilization of one of the ova in the ovary of a developing embryo, so that, a second imperfect individual is formed which is of a later date than the embryo. The impregnation may be regarded as due to surplus spermatozoa remaining near the morula, fertilizing the primordial ovum which is developed early.

(ii) Cell-rest theory :

According to this theory, the cells divide actively and give rise to teratoma.

(iii) Impregnation of the mature ovum before it leaves the graffian-follicle.

Pathology

It is usually unilateral and pedenculated. It is generally unilocular, but may contain 2-3 loculi. Its surface is smooth but yellow in colour. The ovary is flattened and incorporated in the cyst wall or it may be well projected. The cavity contains sebacious (thick jelly-like) material and hair. Projecting into the cavity is a solid part consisting of teeth, liver, bone, cartilages and thyroid gland. All the three layers of embryo being represented, the whole is covered by the skin. The cyst wall is lined by skin near embryoma. In other places, it is smooth or may be covered by granulation tissue with hair and cholestrin plates embedded in it. Granulation tissue is caused by the irritation of hair. It occurs in all ages (even the infants get it) and grows slowly, rarely becoming larger than the foetal head. It is an innocent tumour, but may become malignant. Should rupture occur, implantation growths may be there, but no metastasis occurs. Corpus luteum is present which shows that the ovary is still active and this should make one hesitate before removing the ovaries in bilateral cysts. Torsion of the pedicle may occur and the cyst becomes parasitic; it is liable to suppuration after labour, otherwise it causes no symptoms.

Signs and Symptoms :

The cysts may be unilateral or bilateral. There is no special age incidence as far as ovarian cysts are concerned. The following signs and symptoms are indicative of ovarian cysts :

1. Abdominal swelling.
2. They hardly ever affect the menstrual functions.
3. Pressure symptoms :

   Big tumours lead to embarrassment of respiration and palpitation as a result of pressure upon the diaphragm; bilateral oedema of the feet may be there due to venous obstruction.
4. Urinary symptoms :

   Like frequency of micturition.
5. Bowel symptoms :

   They are, of course, rare because the soft consistence of the cysts is insufficient to obliterate the lumen of the intestines.
6. Pain of dull, dragging and constant nature in one or other iliac fossa ; it is most likely to be due to pressure upon the pelvic organs.
7. Ovarian cachexia may develop in case of large ovarian cysts; then, the patient becomes emaciated.
8. When axial rotation of an ovarian cyst occurs, there is extremely severe abdominal pain, shock and collapse with subnormal temperature and later on distension and constipation, poor abdominal movement, tense and tender cyst.
9. Physical signs :

On inspection : The typical ovarian cyst forms an abdominal swelling, the abdominal wall can be seen to move over the swelling on deep inspiration ; the tumour is symmetrically situated in the abdomen and is not more prominent to one side of the midline.

On Palpation : The upper and lateral limits can be defined but not the lower one usually. The surface of the tumour is smooth ; small cysts are movable from side to side. The consistence of the tumour is tense and cystic and a fluid thrill can be elicited.

Differential Diagnosis :

The abdominal physical signs of an ovarian cyst may be simulated by the following conditions :—

1. Full bladder.
2. Pregnant uterus.
3. Myoma.
4. Ascites.

1. Full Bladder : Full bladder is tense and tender, fixed in position, projecting anteriorly more than an ovarian cyst, and a catheter should be passed to establish the diagnosis. History of retention of urine is important here.

2. Pregnant Uterus : It gives painless uterine contractions felt on the abdomen. The diagnosis can be made by careful bimaanual examination, X-ray and positive biological tests of pregnancy.

3. Myoma : It is usually hard and firm without the tense cystic consistence of the ovarian cyst, it is continuous and movable with the cervix.

4. Ascites : In this condition, shifting dullness and fluid thrill are important.

	Myoma	*Ovarian Cyst*
1.	**Tumour is usually solid and hard.**	**Tumour is cystic.**
2.	**Cervix is usually continuous with it. If we move the body the cervix will move with it.**	**Cervix does not move with the body.**

3. When sound is put into the uterus it moves with the tumour.	There is no such movement.
4. Uterine cavity is enlarged.	No enlargement of the uterine body.
5. Menorrhagia is common.	No menorrhagia.

Ascites	*Ovarian Cyst*
1. Fullness in lumbar regions and flatness in the centre.	Centre is full and lumbar regions are flat.
2. There is no definite outline; the water gravitates to one side or the other.	There is definite outline.
3. There is a thrill by tapping.	No marked thrill.
4. Middle area is resonant; dullness in the flanks.	Dull in the middle and resonant at the flanks.
5. Shifting dullness is noted.	Dullness is fixed.
6. Distance from ensy-form cartilage to umbilicus is more than the distance from umbilicus to pubis.	Distance from umbilicus to pubic is much longer.
7. Distance from umbilicus to the anterior superior iliac spines is equal.	It is longer on one side than the other.

Complications :

1. Abortion.
2. Rupture.

Treatment :

Treatment is generally symptomatic. But, in some cases, bilateral oophorectomy is recommended, particularly, those who do not respond favourably with suitable medicines and those where malignancy is threatened.

Homoeopathic remedies :

Apis, Aurum iod., Colch., Iod., Lyco., Oophorinum, Medo., Thuja, Conium, Lach., Rhod.

TUMOURS OF THE OVARIES

THERAPEUTIC HINTS

Apis : Sudden stitches, like bee-stings, in the tumour, or sharp, cutting pains, with scanty urine and constipation; bearing down, and pain in the small of the back, as if the menses would come on ; numbness of the corresponding lower extremity ; thirstlessness; pale skin; oedema; right side.

Arsenic : Burning pain; restlessness; anxiety; oppression; sinking of strength; great thirst, but little drinking at a time; dropsical swelling all over; pain in the corresponding leg; cannot keep the foot still.

Calc. carb. : Distension and hardness of the abdomen; pressure in the rectum, and bearing down in the womb; profuse and too early menses; obese constitution.

Cantharis : Burning pain ; great sensitiveness of the abdominal walls ; constant, painful urging to urinate and defaecate ; tensemus in the bladder and rectum ; wretched, sickly appearance.

China : After great loss of fluids ; general anasarca ; meteorism.

Colocynth : A firm, elastic tumour occupies the space between the uterus and the vagina anteriorly and the rectum posteriorly, completely occluding the vagina and rendering defaecation very difficult. Paroxysms of acute pain across the hypogastrium, in the sacral region and around the hip joint when attempting to walk ; the pain extends down the groin and along the femoral nerve; it is relieved by flexing the thigh upon the pelvis, and always induced or aggravated by extending the thigh ; but there are frequent and severe paroxysms without any provocation.

Iodium : Pressing, bearing down towards the genitals ; constipation ; acrid leucorrhoea, corroding the parts; dwindling and falling away of the mammae; strumous constitution.

Lilium tig. : Bearing down in the uterine region, worse walking, better holding up the abdomen with the hands; tenderness of the swollen left ovary; stinging, burning pains from ovary up into the abdomen and down the thigh; shooting pains from left ovary across the pubes; urine causes a smarting sensation; prolapsed and sensitive uterus.

Lycopodium : Painful boring stitches in the left ovarian region; pressure on the rectum and bladder; pain in the sacral region, especially when rising from a seat ; red, sandy sediment in the urine; ascites ; varicose veins on the legs.

Plumbum : The patient wants to stretch the upper and lower limbs during ovarian pains.

Podophyllum : Tumour on right side; pain and numbness extending down the corresponding thigh. Pains extend upward to the shoulder.

Stramonium : Tumour attended with some lancinating pains and hysterical convulsions. During the convulsions the patient shrinks back with fear on seeing any one.

In cases where proper homoeopathic treatment fails to show any influence in staying the growth of such tumours, or in improving the general health of the patient, operative surgery (tapping with subsequent iodine injections, electrolysis, ovariotomy) is indicated.

TUMOURS OF THE BREASTS

CHAPTER LI

BENIGN TUMOURS

(a) Fibro-adenoma : hard and soft.

(b) Papilloma

(c) Lipoma.

(a) Fibro-Adenoma : Hard and Soft : The age of occurrence of hard adenoma is 15-30 years. It is highly movable and painless small swelling in the breast tissue. Its development is a slow growing process.

Soft adenoma is a tumour covering larger area. It is not freely movable and grows more rapidly and is seen above the age of 30 years.

Surgical removal provides the only satisfactory treatment.

(b) Papilloma : This is a cherry like tumour felt as a small nodule behind the nipple. In this affection the patient complaints of bleeding from the nipple on pressing.

Removal of the tumour is the recommended treatment.

(c) Lipoma : It means the tumour or the extra growth of the fatty tissue. So, here it denotes an abnormal collection of fat in the breast tissue.

Treatment may be surgical removal of the extra fatty growth or based upon the obese tendency.

CHAPTER LII
MALIGNANT TUMOURS OF THE BREASTS

(a) Cancer of pregnancy and lactation
(b) Medullary carcinoma
(c) Scirrhus variety
(d) Atrophic type
(e) Paget's disease.

(a) Cancer of pregnancy and lactation : It is technically known as Mastitis-carcinosa. Being malignant in nature, the rate of its growth is very rapid. It is seen during pregnancy or lactation The symptoms of redness, tenderness and even temperature may be there but no pus formation though it is apparently an abscess. Blood examination will clear the condition as there is no leucocytosis in cancer.

Treatment :

1. Radio therapy ; but, preferably,
2. Termination of pregnancy, and
3. Removal of the breast tissue.

(b) Medullary carcinoma : This, too, is an affection of the younger age group, below 30 years It is a fast growing but painless growth. The veins under the skin may be congested.

Treatment is the surgical removal of the growth.

(c) Scirrhus variety : It is a painless tumour with a history of one to three years.

(d) Atrophic type : This growth is seen in old aged women having atrophied breasts. The process of development is slow. The most important sign here is the retraction of the nipple to a higher level. We can feel the tumour with the palm. Axillary lymph glands are found to be enlarged. All the findings are, however, to be confirmed by histological examination of the breast tissue.

(e) Pagets disease of the breast : It starts as chronic eczema of the nipple. It eats away the nipple and areola. This process is slowly developing. It is not seen during lactation ; but it is a disease of the old age. Nipple is eaten away and there is no favourable response to the treatment. It is a unilateral affection. All these points will distinguish this condition from eczema of the nipple wherein the symptoms will be just opposite.

Treatment is the removal of the whole breast tissue.

Diagnosis of cancer is through biopsy, of course, because the symptoms are often confusing and may lead to another condition.

TREATMENT :

Treatment of cancer is three fold :

1. Surgery,
2. Radio-therapy, and
3. Hormonal treatment.

Apart from the surgical removal of the breast tissue, sometimes removal of the ovaries proves beneficial.

And above all, the indicated homoeopathic remedies bring about very good results :—

Bufo, Conium, Graph., Silicea, Merc., Hydras., Ars., Calc. iod., Carcinocin, etc.

TUMOURS OF THE BREASTS

THERAPEUTIC HINTS

Conium : This remedy has a specific action on the female breast, removing its engorgements and tumours and relieving its pains. Tumours of a suspicious nature in the mammae have been caused to disappear by the use of Conium. They are the seat of a piercing pain, worse at night, and the rest of the gland is tender. It is also given for injuries of the breast from a blow or pressure or overuse of arms ; the characteristics are the hardness and extreme tenderness ; the breasts are painful even to the touch of clothes or jar of walking. Especially suitable when the gland gets inflamed after every little cold; or if the origin of the tumour can be traced to a bruise. Pruritus is also an accompanying symptom.

Phytolacca : Irritable mammary tumours; fatty tumours as well as hard painful nodosities in the breast. Cancer of the breast, when the tumour is hard, painful and purple. The breasts are very sensitive during nursing, with an excessive flow of milk. There is a tendency of the breast to cake and suppurate ; the pains seem to radiate from the nipple all over the body, especially down the arm from the axilla. Patient is chilly, having rigors indicating suppuration ; sore and fissured nipples. Great aching all over the body.

Arnica : Tumours of the mammary gland from bruises. There is a discolouration of the parts and everything adds to the soreness, such as clothing, bandages, etc.

Apis : When there is stinging, burning pain, whether in scirrhous tumours or in open cancers ; pain in the ovarian region, with bearing down ; scanty, dark urine ; oedema of the lower extremities.

Arsenic : Nightly, burning pain like fire, with great restlessness; loss of strength and emaciation ; the pains grow better from the external application of warmth.

Arsenic iodide : With swelling of gland in axilla.

Asterias rub : Recommended for cancers of the left breast.

Belladonna : Scirrhous tumours, with erysipelatous inflammation and stitching pain ; frequent bearing down in the genital organs.

Bromium : After the extirpation of a hard tumour in the left breast, there appears a hard, uneven tumour in the right breast, which is grown tight to its surroundings ; periodical lancinating pains, especially at night, worse from external pressure; grayish, earthy complexion of the face ; suppression of menses; emaciation and great depression of spirits.

Calc. carb. : Indurations of the breast; too early and too profuse menstruation ; soreness and swelling of breast before the menses.

Calcarea fluor : A routine tissue remedy in the treatment of the tumours. Most useful for knots, kernels, or hardened lumps in the female breast, accompanied with indurated glands of stony hardness. It will prevent the development of cancer in cases where the breasts present suspcious lumps.

Calc. ox. : Has, more than any other remedy, relieved the terrible pains in open cancers.

Carbo an. : Scirrhous tumour, hard and uneven ; the skin over it is loose, on places of a dirty, blue-red appearance ; the pains are burning and drawing toward the axilla; oppression of the chest; nightly perspiration of the thighs only; desponding.

Chim. umb. : Tumour broke and left a small, irregular ulcer, with wasted edges, sloughing, discharging foetid pus ; axillary glands enlarged.

Clematis : Scirrhus, left side, with stitches in the shoulder ; or when the whole gland is very painful, worse in cold weather and during the night ; worse during the growing moon ; while perspiring, she cannot bear to be uncovered.

Graphities : When the tumour grows out of old cicatrices, which have been formed by repeated gatherings of the breast.

Hydrastis : Scirrhous tumour ; hard, heavy, and adhernt to the skin, which is dark, mottled and very much puckered ; the nipple being retracted ; pains like knives thrust into the part; cachectic appearance of the face.

Lachesis : Tumour in the left breast, with lancinating pain; in consequence of pressure upon the tumour the pain extends into the left shoulder and down the arm ; there is a constant painful feeling of weakness and lameness in the left shoulder and arm, which is aggravated by using the arm. In open cancer, when it has a dark, bluish-red appearance, with blackish streaks of coagulated and decomposed blood ; chronic leucorrhoea ; painful menstruation on the first day.

Lapis albus : For cases of incipient scirrhus of the mammary glands, with retraction of the nipple. Many cases of goitre are amenable to the action of this remedy. Also useful for malignant diseases of the uterus where the discharges are black and offensive and intense burning all through the diseased parts.

Lycopodium : Hard tumours, with stitching or cramping pain; circumscribed redness of the face ; worse from 4 P.M. ; during the paroxysms of pain she is obliged to walk about and to weep; she feels better in the open air.

Murex : Given to quiet the pains of mammary tumours, especially when these pains are increased during menses.

Phosphorus : When the ulcer bleeds easily.

Plumbum iod : Inflamed indurated masses in the female breast, slowly developing. The hard unchangeable character, the slow development and the supervention of painful inflammations.

Sepia : Indurations in the breast and ovaries ; yellow, spotted face; chronic leucorrhoea.

Silicea : With great itching of the swollen gland. It often relieves the pains of cancer, lupus and sarcoma with thick yellow and offensive discharge.

Sulphur : One of the best remedies for mammary tumours. Burning is a prominent symptom ; with a history of former skin diseases and suppressed eruptions or of an infective leucorrhoea.

Baryta iod. : Hard cancerous tumours of the breast. Ovarian tumours with a scrofulous taint.

Scrofularia nodosa : Has a special affinity for the breast tissue. Adenoma and carcinoma come within its curative range.

——

DISPLACEMENTS OF THE UTERUS

When the uterus does not maintain the normal position or place in the pelvis, it is called a displaced uterus. Normally the uterus is slightly anterverted and anteflexed. Version refers to the direction of the cervical canal, whereas, flexion refers to the inclination of the body of uterus on the cervix.

The uterine body may get bent making an angle within the cervix at the isthmus or the internal os. It is quite different from the whole of the uterus lying far back or front in the pelvis.

The common displacements of the uterus are as follows :

(i) **Forward displacements :**

(a) Anterversion.

(b) Anteflexion.

(ii) **Backward displacements :**

(a) Retroversion.

(b) Retroflexion.

(iii) **Downward displacements :**

Prolapse :

1st degree : **When cervix descends into the vagina.**

2nd degree : **When cervix descends to the level or vulva.**

3rd degree : **When cervix protrudes outside the vaginal. orifice.**

And when whole of the uterus protrudes outside the vulva, the condition is called complete procedentia.

(iv) **Inversion** :

Here, the uterus turns inside out.

Aetiology :

The displacements are caused by many lapses from the normal conditions such as :—

1. Lack of support or the rupture of perineum.
2. Increased pressure from above by straining, etc.
3. Increased weight of the uterus from sub-involution and after pregnancy.
4. Chronic inflammations and congestions.
5. Traction of adhesions resulting from pelvic cellulitis.
6. Tumours, etc.

——

DISPLACENTS OF THE UTERUS

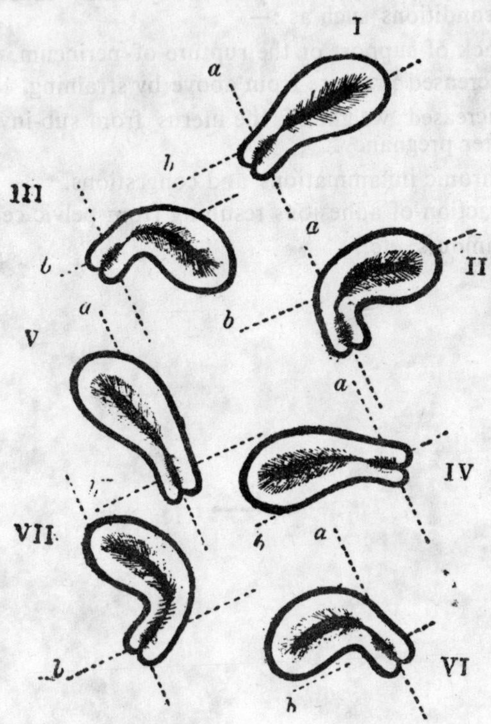

a. Axis of the Vagina ;
b. Axis of the Normal Uterus.
I. Normal Position ;
II. Anteflexion, fundus in Normal position ;
III. Anteflexion, Cervix in Normal Position ;
IV. Retroversion ;
V. Partial Retroversion
VI. Retroversion with Retroflexion ;
VII. Anteversion with Retroflexion.

CHAPTER LIII
RETROVERSION

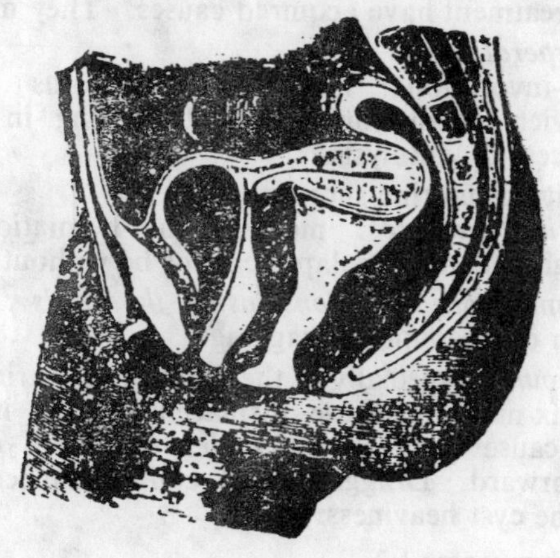

Retroversion of the uterus

RETROVERSION means the backward displacement of the uterus ; i.e., it is tilted back on its own axis.

For the convenience of expression, it has been divided into 3 degrees :

1. First degree of retroversion : In this condition, the fundus lies near the level of 3rd sacral vertebra.

2. Second degree of retroversion : Here the fundus lies in the hollow of the sacrum.

3. Third degree of retroversion : It is said to be there when the fundus lies in the pouch of Douglas.

Aetiology :

The causes have been divided into :—

A. Congenital, and

B. Acquired

A Congenital Causes : They may be due to maldevelopment of the uterus ; but, it is a rare condition.

B. Acquired Causes : Most of the cases coming, now-a-days, for treatment have acquired causes. They may be :

(1) *Puerperal causes* :

(a) Sub-involution : i.e., when the uterus still remains heavier. Involution means decreasing in size by the process of autolysis.

(b) Laxity of uterine support.

(2) *Uterine prolapse :* meaning the herniation of uterus into the vaginal canal. Prolapse cannot be without retroversion.

(3) *Inflammatory adhesions inside the pelvis :* They cause retroversion on account of dragging.

(4) *Tumours* : especially of the uterus and ovaries. Tumours in the cervix may not cause displacement ; but in the fundus, they may cause displacement under the force of heaviness, bending forward. Dragging will cause displacement of the uterus by the cyst heaviness.

Signs and Symptoms :

1. Backache : It is due to strain and stretch on the nerves and congestion in the uterine vessels. On account of tilting of the uterus backwards, the tubes get twisted causing congestion.

2. Menorrhagia and Dysmenorrhoea :—Occurring due to the chronic congestion.

3. Leucorrhoea : As a result of congestion, there is exudate which comes out in the form of leucorrhoeal discharge from the vagina.

4. Sterility :

(i) Due to displacement of the uterus backwards, it causes displacement of the cervix ; it may be away from the seminal pool ; and thus the sperms may not reach the cervix because it lies upwardly.

(ii) Or, there might be twisting of the tubes, so that, there is complete occlusion of the lumen, thereby hindering the passage of the ovum, from the ovaries to the uterus ; for this reason, the conception does not take place.

5. **Dyspareunia** : Pain during the intercourse always shows displaced position of the ovaries ; they are likely to be placed in the pouch of Douglas.

6. **Chronic pain in inguinal region** : On deep pressure, of course.

Physical Exemination :

It is always done bimanually.

1. **Vaginal Examination (P.V.) :** Direction of the cervix is found changed ; its normal position is backward and downward ; but in the third degree of retroversion, it is forward and downward.

2. **Put the finger into the vagina :** and the other hand over the abdomen and palpate the fundus. In the third degree of retroversion, the uterus is palpated in the pounch of Douglas.

3. **Find out the mobility of uterus :** As far as it is mobile, it can be treated with medicines ; but. when it is fixed, it cannot be treated with the medicines ; because great adhesions may have been formed.

4. **On P.V. ezamination :**—Tumours can also be found.

Differential Diagnosis :

1. Sycabalous masses in the rectum, i.e., loaded rectum.
2. Uterine fibroids.
3. Ovarian tumours, lying in the pouch of Douglas.
4. Old pervic haematocele.

1. Sycabalous masses in the rectum :— Hard ball-like stools accumulated int he rectum; so that, on P.V. examination, one may feel something big, thinking that to be retroverted uterus.

(1) It will pit on pressure if exerted on the posterior vaginal wall.

(2) Direction of the cervix is normal.

(3) One can feel the fundus bimanually.

2. *Uterine Fibroids* : The fibroids in the lower uterine segment felt in the pouch of Douglas may be mistaken for retroversion. In this condition, the positions of uterus and cervix are, however, normal.

3. *Ovarian Cyst* : The cyst may be present without causing any displacement of the uterus and ovaries. The uterus may be displaced if the ovaries are displaced.

4. *Pelvic haematocele* : Haematocele is the collection of blood forming a blood tumour. Its characteristics are as follows:-

(1) They are partly solid and partly soft.

(2) Two swellings are felt in the pelvic region : one of haematocele and the other of retroverted uterus. Two swellings connot be the same thing at the same time.

Treatment :

Mostly, the cases are of acquired variety ; and the common cause in them is the puerperal cause. So, preventive treatment is important in the form of proper management in antenatal and postnatal periods.

1. Certain Exercises : They are meant, firstly to bring the uterus back to the normal position and secondly, to tone up the pelvic floor muscles.

(1) Lying in the knee-chest position.

(2) To contract and relax the levator-ani muscles which are lying around the rectum for toning up the pelvic floor muscles.

2. Diet : Vitamins, minerals and proteins ; so that the patient may gain general health.

3. Drugs : Abies can., Aesc. hip., Eupiol, Fraxinus amer., Helonias, Lilium tig., Kreosote, Murex, Podo., Puls., Platina, Stannum, Sepia.

4. Insertion of pessaries and rings : They are to be used for a certain period of time, as long as the patient is being treated.

(1) During early pregnancy to the prevent abortion or incarceration.

(2) In sterility for correction of displāced uterus.

(3) During puerperium : It is also useful after delivery when the uterus has a tendency to fall backward.

(4) For pessary test : It means, to see whether the replacement cures the symptoms.

(5) When the operation is contra-indicated.

Disadvantages of pessaries :

Vaginitis, adhesions and ulceration of the vaginal wall.

Essentials of pessary treatment :

(1) It must keep the uterus in position.
(2) It must not cause any discomfort or any urinary dysfunction.
(3) It should be worn for three months and then removed.

Contra-indications for use of pessary :

(1) Adherent retroversion.
(2) Inflammation of ovaries, tubes and parametrium.
(3) When future medical care is not available.
(4) Tender and prolapsed ovaries.

Pessary-Test

If symptoms recur after removal of the pessary, operational treatment is advised. The patient is tranied to douche with distilled water when the pessary is in its place and if any discharge is occuring.

It is important to replace the uterus before insertion of the pessary.

5. **Surgery** : When pelvic adhesions are formed and when the uterus does not remain mobile, it is not a case of medicines to be treated with.

Surgery is indicated in those cases where the body is not responding to the medicines. There are two such indications.

1. In mobile and uncomplicated retroversion where the symptoms keep on recurring after removal of the pessaries; of course, selected cases of habitual abortion and sterility.
2. Complicated fiixed retroversion with adhesions or prolapse.

CHAPTER LIV
PROLAPSES

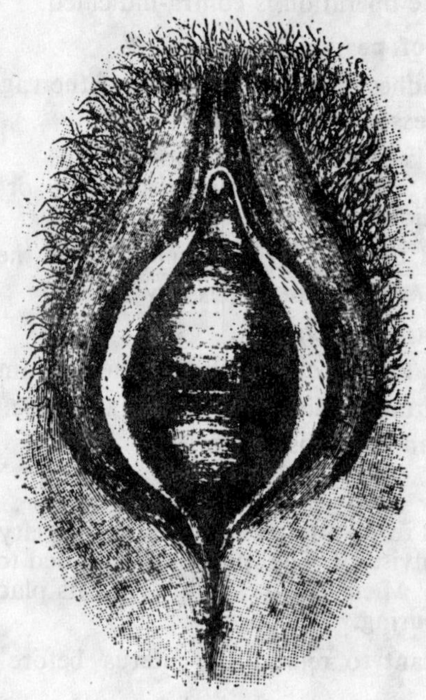

Cystcele and Rectocele.

PROLAPSE is the herniation of the pelvic organs through the vagina.

Types of Prolapses

(i) Cystocele

(ii) Rectocele

(iii) Urethrocele

(iv) Enterocele

(v) Uterine prolapse.

(i) **Cystocele** : It means prolapse of the bladder alongwith the anterior vaginal wall.

(ii) **Rectocele** : It means protrusion of the rectum alongwith the posterior vaginal wall.

(iii) **Urethocele** : It means protrusion of the urethra with the anterior vaginal well.

(iv) **Enterocele** : It is the pouch of Douglas that protrudes alongwith its contents (loops of intestine) into the vagina.

(v) **Uterine Prolapse** : It means protrusion of the uterus into the veginal canal ; alongwith it retroversion must be present.

Clinical Varieties of Uterine Prolapse

(i) **Vagino-Uterine** :—It is prolapse of the vaginal wall dragging the uterus alongwith it.

(ii) **Utero-Vaginal** :—Uterus is retroverted and prolapsing into the vagina dragging the vaginal wall alongwith it ; there is inversion of the vaginal wall.

Degrees of Uterine Prolapse

1. **First degree of Prolapse** : Cervix and whole of the uterus descends from its normal position into the vagina and the external os lies at the level of the ischial spine which means a slight degree of prolapse.

2. **Second degree of Prolapse** : The cervix lies at or outside the vagina (external os).

3. Third Degree of Prolapse

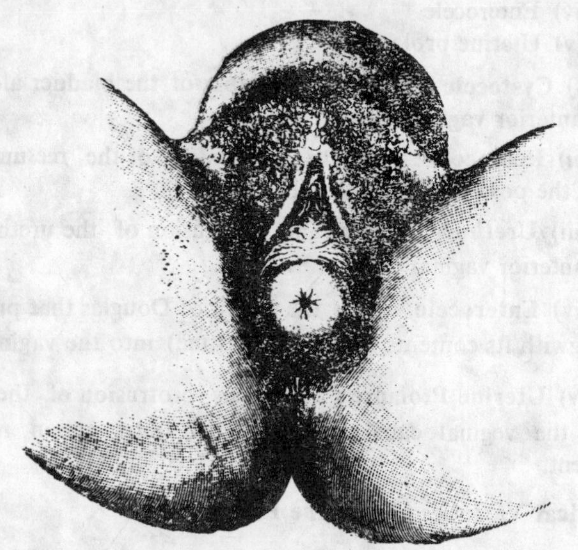

Procedentia of Uterus due to the pressure of two ovarian Dermoids.

The uterus lies outside the vagina : it is called PROCEDENTIA : in it, the uterus is completely inverted (i.e., inside out).

Aetiology :

Causes have been divided under two heads :

1. Laxity and atony of pelvic support.
2. Increased intra-abdominal pressure.

1. Laxity :

A. Congenital of developmental defects : Causing atony of the pelvic floor-but it is a rate condition.

B. Acquired Causes : These are very important. They may be :

(1) Trauma during child birth : Such as, lacerations, perineal tears either by repeated deliveries or instrumental delivery.

(2) **Early bearing down during first stage of labour :—** i.e., when the pains are on and there is no dilatation of the os, the lady should not bear down.

(3) **Delivering baby without emptying the bladder :**

(4) **Improper management during puerperium :** Early ambulation should not be allowed.

(5) **Asthenic atony :** It may be due to menopause or undernutrition before during pregnancy.

2. Increased intra-abdominal presasure

It may occur due to the flowing reasons :

(1) Constipation, acute or chronic.

(2) Chronic severe coughing.

(3) Obesity.

(4) Heavy weight-lifting.

Anything which causes increased intra-uterine pressure may cause prolapse of the uterus.

For the aetilogy of prolapse, one should remember 6 Cs :

Congenital.
Confinement.
Climacteric.
Cough.
Constipation and
Constitution, fat.

Signs And Symptoms

1. Beraing down sensation : Characterisic symptom of prolapse is the bearing down sensation, as if something is protruding out of the vagina.

2. Sacral Backache :— It is due to stretching of the nerves and ligaments and secondly, due to congestion. As the uterus is retroverted, so, there will be twisting of the blood vessels and thus there would be congestion.

3. Leucorrhoea : It occurs due to :

(1) Congestion as a result of twisting of the blocd vessels.

(2) Puerperal infection : cervicitis or vaginitis.

4. Menorrhagia and Metrorrhagia : Menorrhagia due to congestion in the endometrium and metrorrhagia in long standing cases causing ulcertation. It is present in all stages ; and

5. Difficulty in walking in procedentia : Because. the mass is protruding our of vagina.

6. In Cystocele :— Apart from the characteristic signs mentioned above, are added special signs ; e. g.,

(1) Difficulty in micturition.

(2) Frequency of micturition.

(3) Retention of urine whole of urtne does not come out, some of it is retained.

(4) Stressed incontinence : it means dribbling of urine. On account of pain, the woman is afraid to pass the urine ; so, it dribbles.

In cystocele, the bladder symptoms are more marked than the uterine symptoms.

7. In Rectocele :—Apart from the above symptoms, are also present :

(1) Difficulty and obstruction of the stools, and

(2) Constipation.

Here, bearing down sensation, sacral backache, leucorrhoea etc. are less marked and the rectal symptoms are more marked.

Diagnosis

1. Age : Incidence of prolapse is common in multipara-menopausal age or child bearing age.

2. Constitutions : These patients are usually of asthenic type or of obese type. In obese type, there is flabby abdomen and the muscles and ligaments are weak.

3. Physical Examination (P. V.) :

(i) In Cystocele : Bulge is felt at the upper part of the anterior vaginal wall.

(ii) In Urethrocele : Bulge is felt at the lower part of the anterior vaginal wall.

(iii) In Rectocele : Bulge is felt at the middle portion of the posterior vaginal wall.

(iv) **In Enterocele** : Bulge is felt at the upper portion of the posterior vaginal wall.

Complications :

(i) **Chronic Invalidism** : Because, the condition is of very long standing nature, the patient cannot walk very much.

(ii) **Renal Failure** : As the urine is retained in the bladdder, it goes back to the kidneys ; so, it produces **Hydronephrosis** or **Pyelonephritis** and even **Renal Failure**.

(iii) **Pelvic Sepsis** : Because there are ulcers present in the cervix, the infection may spread to the pelvic floor, causing pelvic abscess.

Treatment

Preventive :—Proper management in ante-natal and post-natal periods ; e.g., avoidance of any illness of the pelvic organs and proper feeding of the mother to avoid anaemia.

Proper management at the time of labour e.g., avoidance of perineal tears, etc. and after labour also, such as, early ambulation, early labour, too many pregnancies, etc.

2. **Curative** :—The principle of treatment is to treat the cause first. Diet is the most important factor. In obese patients, cut down the proteins, whereas in asthenic patients, feed with more proteins.

Homoeopathic remedies :

Aletris farinosa, Aloe, Cauloph., Calc. carb., Collinsonia, Fraxinus americana, Helon., Lil. tig., Platina, Podo., Puls., Sepia, Stannum, Trillium, Graph., Phyto., Fucus ves., Calc. phos., Phos., Silicea.

3. **Exercises and Pessaries** :—These have to be advised to bring the uterus to normal position.

4. **Surgery** :—There are, however, cases which cannot be cured with the medicines ; they shall have to be sent to the surgeon for the repair of the pelvic floor.

CHAPTER LV
INVERSION

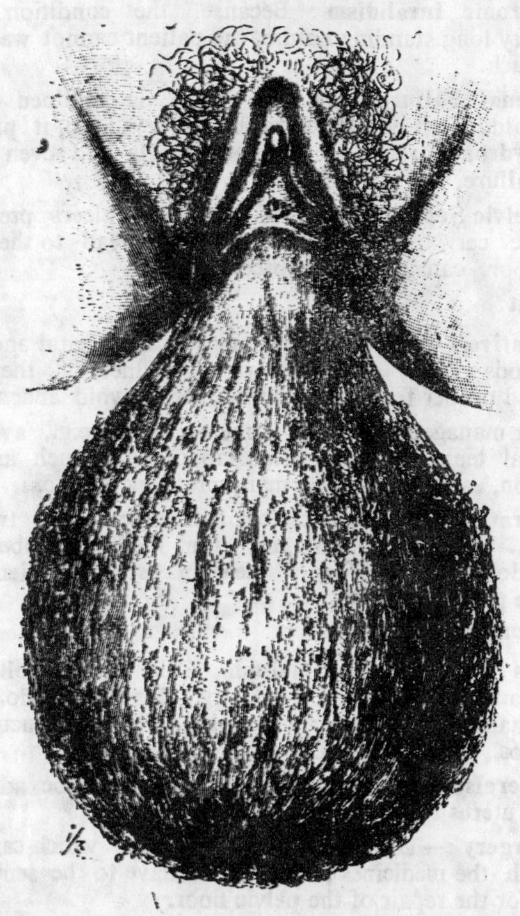

Inversion of the uterus and vagina. The dark spot on each side indicates the Orifice of the fallopian tube.

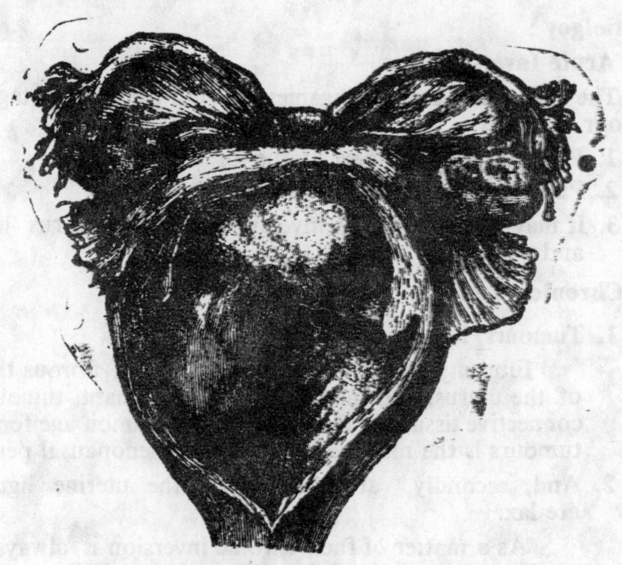

Partial inversion of a uterus due to a Fibroid.

When the uterus is turned inside out, whether partly or wholly, it is known as INVERSION. (Prolapse is the descending of uterus, as it is)

Varieties :

1. Complete inversion, and
2. Incomplete inversion.

When the uterus comes out wholly, it is complete inversion. In it, whole of the uterus, including the cervix, is inverted.

In the incomplete variety, only the fundus protrudes through the cervix.

3. Acute inversion, and
4. Chronic inversion.

Acute inversion is of obstetrical and emergency variety. It is also known as puerperal inversion.

Aetiolgoy :

Of Acute Inversion :

The causes are bad management during the third stage of labour : such as.

1. Pressing upon an inert uterus, or
2. Pulling upon the umbilical cord, or
3. It may be spontaneous inversion when the uterus is lax and placenta is attached.

of Chronic Inversion :

1. Tumours, like fibromyoma or sarcoma.

   Fibromyoma is the benign tumour of fibrous tissues of the uterus; and sarcoma is the malignant tumour of connective tissues of the uterus. The common age for such tumours is the menopausal and post menopausal periods.

2. And, secondly, at that period, the uterine ligments are lax.

   As a matter of fact, chronic inversion is always due to the extra growth of the uterus.

Signs and Symptoms :

Acute Inversion :

It is an emergency condition ; so, the cardinal signs and symptoms of acute inversion are :

I. Shock :

Pallor, air-hunger, cold sweats, rising pulse rate and falling blood pressure, pulse becoming feeble and fast, etc.

2. Bleeding, and
3. Appearance of swelling at the vulva.

Prognosis, here is, of course, grave.

Chronic Inversion :

1. Bearing down pains.
2. Backache.
3. Blood stained discharge.
4. Difficulty in micturition due to obstruction by the pressure of the uterus on the anterior vaginal wall.

5. Anaemia, and
6. General weakess.

Physical Examination (in chronic inversion).

Physical examination, here, contsists of P. V., abdominal and rectal examinations.

On P. V. : A mass is felt protruding out of the cervix.

On Abdominal Examination : (It is done for detecting the position of fundus). A depression at the place will be noticed where fundus should have been present.

Incomplete inverson :

1. The fundus is felt by the finger just above the internal os, because it is protruding out.
2. Cervical rim is felt.
3. If a uterine sound is passed, it can pass through the cervix.

Complete Inversion :

1. Cervical rim is not felt.
2. Swelling is felt in the vagina itself.
3. Sound cannot pass through the cervix.

Differential Diagnosis :

The inversion should be differentially diagnosed from tumours :

Fibroids at the os and

Carcinoma of the cervix.

Fibroids at the os :

1. Fundus is felt at its proper place on abdominal examination.
2. Uterine sound can be passed to the normal distance of the uterus.

   (Normal distance is 3″ from the external os and 4″ to $4\frac{1}{2}$″ is the length of vagina).

Carcinoma of cervix :

I. The fundus is felt at its proper place on abdominal examination.

2. Uterine sound can be passed to the normal distance of the uterus.
3. Cauliflower like growth at the cervix with a history of bleeding on touch, especially at the time of P. V. examination and intercourse.

Treatment :

1. Important thing is to Treat Anaemia and improve the general health of the patient.
2. **Replacement** by Aveling's repositor (a cup shaped instrument).

Remedies :

Aur. mur. nat., Phos., Sepia, Thuja, Fucus vesiculosus, Phytolacca, Silicea, Calcereas, Graphites, etc.

4. If all fail, **Operative Removal** of the uterus, especially in old women, where the fibroid condition is present, is to be done.

Partial or comlete hysterectomy through vaginal route or abdominal opening is advised

---

DISPLACEMENTS OF UTERUS

THERAPEUTIC HINTS

Dr. Kent's views about the pessary treatment :

"It is a common practice to apply a support to hold in position a displaced uterus and then begin to build up by medicine. Who is wise enough to know what to administer after the symptoms, the only true expression of disease, have been removed ! Yet, this is the way some of our specialists go about it, and then complain that "the law is failure." There might be some reason in first taking the symptoms by which to select a remedy and then applying a pessary ; but, to the experienced, the folly of this will appear, as it is so well known that the symptoms immediately disappear without mechanics. Support is not needed after the right remedy has been taken for two days. Again, if a support be used, one has no evidence of good or bad seletion. The cure of these diseases is possible without support with pure medicinal treatment."

Aconite : After a sudden fright ; also when inflammatory symptoms prevail. Agonizing pain during the menses, with tossing about. Fear of death.

Aesculus hipp : Inflamed cervix uteri, retroversion, prolapse, enlargement and induration, when charaterised by great tenderness, heat, throbbing, piles—mostly blind, and pain and stiffness of the back.

Agaricus muscarius : Prolapsus after cessation of menses ; bearing—down pain, almost intolerable.

Ammon mur : Pain as from sprain in the groin, obliging one to walk crooked ; menses appear too soon, with pain in the belly and small of the back ; they flow more abundantly in the night; discharge of quantity of blood with the stool during the catamenia.

Arctium lappa : Especially in old cases of prolapsus and procedntia.

Alstonia constricta : (1) Great debility, with loos of appetite from weak digestion. Tongue generally coated a dirty white, aggravated on toward the base, although it may be clean.

Debility, dependent on a lack of digestive power of stomach or assimilative power of system. Not in debility of nervous type, or in consequence of lagrippe.

(2) Menses, aggravated mornings before breakfast, or at irregular times especially when depending or reflex irrigation from pelvic organs.

(3) An empty, gone feeling in stomach or else in the whole abdomen, coming at irregular times, with bearing and dragging down sensation in the hypogastrium.

Argentum met : Pain in the small of the back, which extends towards the front and downwards; pain in the left ovary and loins.

Argum niricum : Prolapsus, with ulceration of os or cervix uteri; painful coition, with bleeding from vagina.

Arnica : After a bruise or concussion, which leaves a bruised and sore feeling in the lower part of the abdomen, so that she cannot walk erect.

Aurum : After lifting a heavy load, a sense of weight in the pelvis, with ischuria and constipation, worse at each menstrual period; great dejection of spirits; longing for death, increasing to a desire for self-destruction; or vehement, the least contradiction excites her wrath.

Belladonna : Pressing early in the morning as if all the contents of the abdomen would issue through the genital organs; drawing pain in the small of the back downwards; flow of blood between the periods ; great dryness of the vagina; frequent, unsuccessful desire to urinate or to evacuate the bowels; only a few drops of urine are discharged from the bladder; and some mucus from the rectum; the uterus comes down when straining at stool; or while urinating, and rises again on walking about back; aches as if it would break; dizziness; roaring in the ears; congestion to the head.

Calc. carb : Pressing on the uterus; aching of the vagina; stinging in the os uteri; the menses appear too soon, and are too profuse; milk-like leucorrhoea; inclination to perspire early about the head, great liability to strain a part by lifting; easily tired by bodily exertions; in walking up stairs she feels dizzy and entirely exhausted; even talking makes her weak;

great inclination to sigh; she cannot get her breath long enough; great susceptibility to catch cold; the feet feel most of the time damp and cold, or else the sole of the feet are burning hot; great desire for hard boiled eggs; big-belliedness; scrofulous diathesis.

Calc. phos. : Every cold causes pains in the joints, and in other places where the bones unite and form a symphysis or suture.

Caulophyllum : Retroversion; menstrual colic; congestion and irritability of uterus; leucorrhoea profuse, muocus.

Chamomilla : Abortus; colicky pain and bearing down, with frequent desire to urinate; frequent discharge of coagulated blood, with tearing pains in the veins of the legs; and violent labour pains in the uterus; she is inclined to be quarrelsome and angry; can hardly stop talking about old vexation things.

China : General weakness in consequence of loss of vital fluids, either by haemorrhages, profuse diarrhoea, or debilitating illness; great disposition to sweat during motion and sleep; feels worse from exposure to the slightest current of air; all pains are worse from slightest touch.

Conium : Pain in the mammae before the menses; pressure from above downwards, and drawing in the legs during the menses; feeble or suppressed menses, sterility; smarting, excoriating leucorrhoea; the flow of urine suddenly stops; cough during pregnancy; cough worse at night, and when lying down; vartigo, worse when lying down, or looking round, or going down stair; indurations in the mammae or other glands.

Ferrum iodide :—Retroversion and consequent pressure upon the rectum, that she can neither stand nor walk; constant tenesmus, with frequent white slimy stools; scanty, deep-coloured urine ; nervous and hysteric spasms; scrofulous diathesis.

Helonias :—Displacement low down ; fundus tilted forward; finger passed with difficulty between os and rectum ; in weak patients.

Hydrastis :—Nosebleed before menses ; backache and headache before and during menses ; discharge like white of egg after menses for ten days with great sexual desire, although coition is painful ; after these ten days follows acrid, corroding leucorrhoea with great irritableness and aversion to coition; at times profuse discharge of hot water from the womb. Constant desire to pass water, with relief after passing it; constipation, dry, lumpy faeces are followed by a matter like white of egg. After eating, regurgitation of food by the mouthful without nausea, with nervousness, irritability and headache ; epigastric region tender to touch and a feeling as of a tight band around the waist, worse at night than in the morning ; cannot sleep until after midnight. Prolapsus uteri with indurated os.

Ignatia :—Violent crampy pressing in the region of the uterus, resembling labour-pains, followed by a purulent, corrosive leucorrhoea ; the menses are scanty, black and of a putrid odour ; she seeks to be alone, is brooding to herself and full of grief ; all her pains are aggravated by drinking coffee or smelling tobacco smoke ; gone feeling in pit of stomach.

Kali carb :—Pain in the small of the back, as though it were pressed in from both sides, with labour-like colic and leucorrhoea ; also during the menses ; the pains in the bowels are apt to recur about 3 O'clock every morning ; bloated face in the morning, especially between the eyebrows and upper lids ; great dryness and itchiness of the skin ; great tendency to start when being slightly touched.

Lachesis : Just as patients with a Lachesis sore throat cannot bear anything touching their neck, so do women afflicted with womb disease constantly pull their dress from off the abdomen ; violent labour-like pressing from the loins downwards during the menses, which are scanty ; palpitation of the heart with numbness in the left arm ; constant feeling of something in the throat which she cannot swallow down ; feeling of a ball rolling in the throat which she cannot swallow down; feeling of a ball rolling in the bladder or abdomen, or in both places ; climacteric period.

Lilium tig. :—Feels as though she would drop as under, must press with hand against vulva ; worse on standing and sometimes when recumbent ; frequent ineffectual urging to urinate and defaecate. Menses scanty, flowing only as long as she is moving about ; leucorrhoea profuse and corroding ; she feels always in a hurry, yet cannot accomplish anything.

Lycopodium :--Chronic dryness of the vagina ; pressing through the vagina on stooping ; chronic suppression of the menses after fright ; incarcerated flatulence ; varicose on the lower extremities ; jerking and twitching of single limbs or of the whole body, sleeping or waking ; always wakes up very cross.

Mecurius :—Peculiar weak feeling in the abdomen, as though she had to hold it up ; close above the genital organs a sensation as if something heavy were pulling downward, accompanied by a pulling pain in both thighs, as if the muscles and tendons were too short. During the menses red tongue, with dark spots and burning ; salt taste in the mouth ; sickly colour of the gums, and the teeth are set on edge ; great tendency to perspire ; all the symptoms worse at night ; inexpressible feeling of some internal, insupportable illness.

Murex :—Very much conscious of the uterus. Feeling as if something was pressing on a sore spot in the pelvis, worse sitting. Pain from right side of the womb to right or left breast. Nymphomania ; least contact or touch of parts causes violent sexual excitement. Sore pain in the uterus. Feeling of protrusion. Prolapse, enlargement of uterus with pelvic tenesums and sharp pains extending towards the breasts, worse by lying down. Dysmenorrhoea and chronic endometritis with displacement. Must keep legs tightly crossed. Leucorrhoea green or bloody ; alternate with mental symptoms, like great sadness, anxiety and dread and aching in sacrum.

Natrum mur :—Pressing and pushing from the side of the abdomen towards the genital organs early in the morning, she has to sit down to prevent a prolapus uteri ; dryness of the vagina and painful embrace ; burning and cutting in the urethra after micturition ; headache on waking every morning; faint, weak voice, and exhaustion from talking; after abuse of quinine, or the local application of nitrate of silver.

Nitric acid :—Violent pressing in the hypogastrium, as if everything were coming out at the pudendum, with pain in the small of the back, through the hips and down the thighs ; she feels so weak that she loses breath and speech. Inclined to looseness of the bowels ; most violent, cutting pain after an evacuation, lasting for hours ; she feels, on the whole, better when riding in a carriage.

Nux vomica :—Prolapsus after straining by lifting, or after miscarriage; constant, painful pressing and burning in the uterine region ; pressive pain in the small of the back, worse when turning in bed ; drawing in the thighs ; constant, unsuccessful urging to stool and constant desire to urinate ; the patient wakes after midnight and lies awake for hours, then falls into a heavy sleep again, constantly dreaming until late in the morning, when she feels disinclined to rise. Always the first remedy after allopathic drugging.

Platina :—Great heaviness, pressing in the genitals, extending through the groins as far as the small of the back ; profuse menses ; great sensitiveness of the parts, with pressing from above down ; internal chilliness and external coldness ; constipation ; feeling of numbness and rigidity here and there ; also with trembling and palpitation of the heart ; haughty disposition.

Podophyllum :—Prolapse from overlifting or straining and often parturition ; great constiveness ; frequent micturition ; weakness and soreness of back especially after washing ; prolapsus ani.

Pulsatilla :—Chilliness and paleness of face ; bad taste in the morning and dry tongue without thirst ; is easily moved to tears.

Rhus tox. :—After a strain of hard labour ; she feels worse after any long walk ; the pain in the small of the back is relieved by lying on hard couch.

Secale cor. :—After parturition ; weakly, thin women.

Sepia :—Pressing in the uterus, oppressing the breathing, from above downwards, as if everything would come out of the vagina, accompanied with colic ; she has to cross her limbs to prevent it, followed by a discharge of jelly-like leucorrhoea ; sense of weight in the rectum not relieved after stool, slow and difficult evacuation from the bowels, although the excrements are soft ; pot-belliedness ; yellow saddle across the bridge of the nose ; gone feeling in the pit of the stomach great weakness, tiredness, despondency and disinclination to move.

Sulphur :—Weak feeling in the genital organs and pressure on the parts ; troublesome itching of the pudendum, with pimples all around and burning in the vagina ; she was scarcely able to sit still ; the menstrual blood is thick, black, and so acrid that it makes the thighs sore ; burning and smarting leucorrhoea ; sudden, imperative urging to urinate to prevent an involuntary flow ; weak fainting, between 11 and 12 A.M., must have something to eat ; restless and sleepless nights ; or a heavy sleep which exhausts her ; heat on the top of head with cold feet ; always feels too hot, especially her feet, which compels her to put them from under the cover; walks stooping ; all the symptoms worse while standing ; psoric diathesis.

Veratruma lbum :—After great fear or fright, with cold sweat, exhausting vomiting and diarrhoea.

Zincum :—Usually feels best during menses ; fidgety of feet.

———